IVF in the Medically Complicated Patient

REPRODUCTIVE MEDICINE AND ASSISTED REPRODUCTIVE TECHNIQUES SERIES

David Gardner
University of Melbourne, Australia

Zeev Shoham
Kaplan Hospital, Rehovot, Israel

Kay Elder, Jacques Cohen
Human Preimplantation Embryo Selection, ISBN: 9780415399739

Michael Tucker, Juergen Liebermann
Vitrification in Assisted Reproduction, ISBN: 9780415408820

John D Aplin, Asgerally T Fazleabas, Stanley R Glasser, Linda C Giudice
The Endometrium, Second Edition, ISBN: 9780415385831

Nick Macklon, Ian Greer, Eric Steegers
Textbook of Periconceptional Medicine, ISBN: 9780415458924

Andrea Borini, Giovanni Coticchio
Preservation of Human Oocytes, ISBN: 9780415476799

Steven R Bayer, Michael M Alper, Alan S Penzias
The Boston IVF Handbook of Infertility, Third Edition, ISBN: 9781841848105

Ben Cohlen, Willem Ombelet
Intra-Uterine Insemination: Evidence-Based Guidelines for Daily Practice, ISBN: 9781841849881

Adam H. Balen
Infertility in Practice, Fourth Edition, ISBN: 9781841848495

Nick Macklon
IVF in the Medically Complicated Patient, Second Edition: A Guide to Management, ISBN: 9781482206692

IVF in the Medically Complicated Patient

Second Edition

A Guide to Management

Edited by

Nick S Macklon, MB ChB, MD, FRCOG
Professor of Obstetrics and Gynaecology, Academic Unit of Human
Development and Health / Faculty of Medicine, University of Southampton,
and Director, Complete Fertility Centre Southampton, Princess Anne
Hospital, Southampton, UK

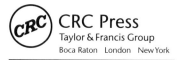

CRC Press
Taylor & Francis Group
Boca Raton London New York

CRC Press is an imprint of the
Taylor & Francis Group, an **informa** business

CRC Press
Taylor & Francis Group
6000 Broken Sound Parkway NW, Suite 300
Boca Raton, FL 33487-2742

© 2014 by Taylor & Francis Group, LLC
CRC Press is an imprint of Taylor & Francis Group, an Informa business

No claim to original U.S. Government works

Printed on acid-free paper
Version Date: 20140304

International Standard Book Number-13: 978-1-4822-0669-2 (Paperback)

Library of Congress Cataloging-in-Publication Data

IVF in the medically complicated patient : a guide to management / editor, Nick S. Macklon. -- Second edition.
    p. ; cm. -- (Reproductive medicine and assisted reproductive techniques series)
    In vitro fertilization in the medically complicated patient
    Includes bibliographical references and index.
    ISBN 978-1-4822-0669-2 (pbk. : alk. paper)
    I. Macklon, Nick S., editor. II. Title: In vitro fertilization in the medically complicated patient. III. Series: Reproductive medicine & assisted reproductive techniques series.
    [DNLM: 1. Fertilization in Vitro--contraindications. 2. Infertility--complications. WQ 208]

RG135
618.1'780599--dc23   2014007812

Visit the Taylor & Francis Web site at
http://www.taylorandfrancis.com

and the CRC Press Web site at
http://www.crcpress.com

Contents

Contributors

JG Al Hashash
Division of Gastroenterology,
   Hepatology and Nutrition
University of Pittsburgh Medical
   Center
Pittsburgh, Pennsylvania, United
   States

AN Andersen
The Fertility Clinic
Copenhagen University Hospital
Rigshospitalet, Copenhagen, Denmark

RA Anderson
MRC Centre for Reproductive Health
University of Edinburgh
Queens Medical Research Institute
Edinburgh, United Kingdom

J Bellver
Department of Obstetrics and
   Gynecology
Faculty of Medicine
University of Valencia and Instituto
   Valenciano de Infertilidad
Valencia, Spain

B Borgström
Department of Clinical
   Science, Intervention and
   Technology
Karolinska Institutet
Karolinska University Hospital
   Huddinge
Stockholm, Sweden

E Campbell
Department of Neurosciences
Belfast Health and Social Care Trust
Belfast, United Kingdom

Y Cheong
Academic Unit of Human Development
   and Health
Faculty of Medicine
University of Southampton
Complete Fertility Centre
   Southampton
Princess Anne Hospital
Southampton, United Kingdom

MA Coleman
University Hospitals
Southampton NHS Foundation Trust
Southampton, United Kingdom

J Craig
Department of Neurosciences
Belfast Health and Social Care Trust
Belfast, United Kingdom

SMC De Sousa
Royal Adelaide Hospital
Adelaide, South Australia, Australia

D Galliano
Department of Reproduction
Instituto Valenciano de Infertilidad
Barcelona, Spain

WL Gianotten
Department of Medical Sexology
University Medical Center
Utrecht, the Netherlands

AJ Goverde
Department of Obstetrics and
   Gynaecology
University Medical Center
Utrecht, the Netherlands

T Hardy
Royal Hospital for Women
Randwick, New South Wales, Australia

PK Heinonen
School of Medicine
University of Tampere and
Department of Obstetrics and
    Gynecology
Tampere University Hospital
Tampere, Finland

O Hovatta
Department of Clinical Science,
    Intervention and Technology
Karolinska Institutet
Karolinska University Hospital
    Huddinge
Stockholm, Sweden

SV Kane
Department of Gastroenterology
Mayo Clinic
Rochester, Minnesota, United States

Y Khalaf
The Assisted Conception Unit
Guy's Hospital
London, United Kingdom

M Krog
The Fertility Clinic
Copenhagen University Hospital
Rigshospitalet
Copenhagen, Denmark

MP Lauritsen
The Fertility Clinic
Copenhagen University Hospital
Rigshospitalet
Copenhagen, Denmark

W Ledger
Department of Obstetrics and
    Gynaecology
School of Women's and Children's Health
University of New South Wales
Sydney, New South Wales, Australia

JG Lemmen
Fertility Clinic Rigshospitalet
Copenhagen, Denmark

A Loft
Fertility Clinic Rigshospitalet
Copenhagen, Denmark

NS Macklon
Academic Unit of Human Development
    and Health
Faculty of Medicine
University of Southampton
Complete Fertility Centre Southampton
Princess Anne Hospital
Southampton, United Kingdom

RJ Norman
The Robinson Institute
School of Pediatrics and Reproductive
    Health
University of Adelaide
Adelaide, South Australia, Australia

GCML Page-Christiaens
Department Obstetrics and Gynaecology
University Medical Center
Utrecht, the Netherlands

A Pellicer
Department of Obstetrics and
    Gynecology
Faculty of Medicine
University of Valencia and Instituto
    Valenciano de Infertilidad
Valencia, Spain

MV Sauer
Department of Obstetrics and
    Gynecology
Columbia University
New York, New York, United States

KT Schmidt
Fertility Clinic
University Hospital of Copenhagen
Rigshospitalet
Copenhagen, Denmark

A Strandell
Department of Obstetrics and
    Gynecology
Sahlgrenska University Hospital
Göteborg, Sweden

SK Sunkara
The Assisted Conception Unit
Guy's Hospital
London, United Kingdom

F Teding van Berkhout
Department of Respiratory Medicine
University Medical Center
Utrecht, the Netherlands

H Tijani
Complete Fertility Centre
    Southampton
Princess Anne Hospital
Southampton, United Kingdom

BB van Rijn
Academic Unit of Human Development
    and Health
University of Southampton
Southampton, United Kingdom

S Ziebe
Fertility Clinic Rigshospitalet
Copenhagen, Denmark

1

The Patient with Cystic Fibrosis

GCML Page-Christiaens, AJ Goverde, and F Teding van Berkhout

CONTENTS

KEY WORDS: *cystic fibrosis, fertility, assisted reproduction, pregnancy*

Introduction

Centralized care in dedicated centres, advances in antibiotic therapy, better nutritional support, and improved treatment of complications have resulted in a considerable improvement of health and life expectancy in both men and women with cystic fibrosis (CF).[1–3] In 2011 the median survival of CF patients in the United States and Canada was 37 years. In observational cohort studies, early diagnosis of CF through neonatal screening was associated with better nutritional status during the first years of life,[4] later colonization with *Pseudomonas aeruginosa*, better lung function at the age of transfer to adult care and increased survival at age 25.[5] The Cystic Fibrosis Foundation Patient Registry 2011 reported that 39.5% of CF patients are married.[3] CF has hence evolved from a paediatric disease to an adult disease. Pregnancy and parenthood may have become a realistic option for some women. However CF does remain a severe chronic disease with limited survival. This chapter addresses the issues relevant to make the best shared decision when women with CF ask for reproductive advice and help.

Background

Epidemiology

In the European Union CF occurs on average in 1 of 4700 liveborns.[6] The Republic of Ireland is an outlier with 1 in 1353, as well as Finland with 1 in 25,000.[2,6] In non-Caucasians the birth incidence is much lower, with 1 in 15,000 newborns affected in North American African Americans and 1 in 31,000 in Asian Americans.[7] In France[8] and in the United States[9] a gradual decrease in birth incidence was noticed during the last two decades, ascribed in part to the fact that preconception, prenatal and newborn screening timely increase the reproductive options of parents at a 1-in-4 risk for a child with CF. Similarly, in the Netherlands a decrease in birth incidence from 1/3600 between 1961 and 1965 to 1/4750 between 1974 and 1994 was reported. Neonatal screening for CF was introduced in the Netherlands in 2011. Immigration from countries with a lower carrier frequency and increased use of prenatal diagnosis and termination of pregnancy in case of an affected fetus have at least in part been held responsible for this decrease.[2]

Pathophysiology

CF is a Mendelian recessive genetic disorder. The normal CF gene on chromosome 7 encodes for the CFTR protein (CF transmembrane conductance regulator gene). CF is caused by mutations in this gene.[10-12] The mutation spectrum and frequency are highly dependent on ethnic origin. More than 1800 CFTR mutations have been identified, the F508del mutation being the most common. The CFTR protein is a chloride channel in the apical membrane of exocrine epithelial cells. In CF this channel is absent, non-functional or deficient. This leads to an imbalance of water and electrolyte movement across the epithelial membrane and thickened secretions, ultimately leading to irreversible organ damage. The lungs and the pancreas are the main affected organs but also other systems such as the reproductive tract can be involved. Several classes of CF mutations have been identified.[13-17] They are described in Table 1.1 and Figure 1.1. In mutation classes I, II and III, no functional CFTR is present in the apical membrane of the epithelium. These mutations lead to more severe CF, with more severe lung disease and pancreatic exocrine insufficiency. Progressive destruction of pancreatic tissue leads to loss of beta cells, causing diabetes. In mutation classes IV and V some residual CFTR activity is present, leading to milder disease with fewer respiratory symptoms, a better nutritional condition and no pancreatic insufficiency.[18]

TABLE 1.1

Classification of CFTR Mutations

Class	Mutations
I	W1282X, G542X, R553X, E822X
II	F508del, D1507, S549I, G85E
III	G551D, S492F, R553G, R560S
IV	R117H, R117C, R117P, L88S
V	3849 + 10kb C→T, 1811 + 1.6kb A→G
	3272-26A→G.

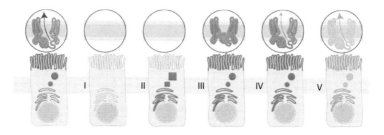

Protein	Normal	Synthesis defect	Folding defect	Regulation defect	Conducting defect	Less CFTR protein
Mutation		G542X	F508del	G551D	R117H	A455E

FIGURE 1.1 Classification of CFTR mutations. In class I and II mutations there is no CFTR protein in the apical membrane. In class III mutations CFTR is present in the cell membrane, but this channel cannot be opened and chloride secretion is therefore absent. In class IV mutations the chloride conduction is diminished and CFTR secretion diminished, and in class V mutations the CFTR production is diminished. (Adapted from Heijerman HGM, De Jonge HR. Ned Tijdschr Geneeskd 2004;148(17):816–9. With permission from the publisher.)

The disturbed water and electrolyte transport also causes problems in other organs, such as obliteration of ductus deferentes (CBAVD, or congenital bilateral absence vas deferens) in male CF patients and viscous cervical mucus in CF females.

Genetics, Genotype-Phenotype Correlations and Modifying Genes

Not only mutations in the CFTR gene but also modifying genes localized outside the CFTR gene and environmental factors determine the severity of lung disease and the occurrence of CF-related complications.

Mutations in CFTR Genes

Most CF patients are homozygotes for severe CFTR gene mutations (predominantly F508del) or compound heterozygotes for severe mutations (for example F508del/G551D). About 10% of CFTR gene mutations are mild (for example F508del/A455E). CF patients without residual CFTR function are prone to develop complications such as meconium ileus (MI), CF-related diabetes (CFRD) and severe CF liver disease with portal hypertension (CFLD). However not all patients with severe CF gene mutations develop these complications. Only 20% of CF neonates are affected by MI, and only 2–5% of adolescent/adult CF patients suffer from severe CFLD. Even among CF patients who are F508del homozygotes and their siblings, lung disease severity varies substantially. This variability in clinical manifestations and severity of disease is caused by modifying genes and environmental factors.

Modifying Genes Outside the CFTR Genes

Case control (association) studies and family-based (linkage) studies have led to the discovery of modifying genes. Most studies were performed in monozygous twins, dizygous twins and non-twin affected siblings.

Lung disease modifying genes: These are mannose-binding lectin 2 (MBL2), endothelial receptor type A (EDNRA) and transforming growth factor beta 1 (TGF-beta 1).[19] Genetic variations in all 3 are associated with lung disease severity or risk of infection with *Pseudomonas aeruginosa*.

Meconium ileus (MI): In CF patients without residual CFTR function, only 20% of patients suffer from MI. CF family studies demonstrated a strong hereditary pattern in the occurrence of MI, but hitherto no modifying genes contributing to the manifestation of MI are known.

CF-related diabetes (CFRD): About 20% of adolescent CF patients suffer from CFRD. This figure rises to 50% in adulthood. In patients with relatives with type 2 diabetes CFRD develops at a younger age.

CF liver disease with portal hypertension (CFLD): This is an infrequent complication in CF patients without CFTR function. It is strongly associated with the Z-allele of the alfa 1-antiprotease (SERPINA 1) gene.

In summary:

- CF mutations without residual CFTR function lead to pancreatic insufficiency, malnutrition and more severe lung disease.
- CF patients with residual CFTR function are pancreatic sufficient and manifest milder lung disease.
- CFTR-deficient CF patients are prone to several complications: meconium ileus, CFRD, CFLD.
- The occurrence of these complications and the variance in severity of lung disease are influenced by modifying genes.
- There are limited data on the relation between genotype and fertility and reproductive outcome.

Clinical Aspects

Cystic fibrosis is a multi-organ disorder. The main clinical manifestations and their therapeutic approach are listed in Table 1.2. Disease variability is determined not only by mutation class and modifier genes as mentioned but also by environmental influences such as nutrition, micro-organisms, tobacco, stress, socio-economic status, time of

TABLE 1.2

Frequently Occurring Problems and Their Management in Patients Suffering from Cystic Fibrosis

Organ System	Symptoms/Syndromes	Therapeutic Measures

Respiratory system	Recurrent bacterial infections
	Bronchiectasis
	Hemoptysis
	Pneumothorax
	Allergic bronchopulmonary aspergillosis
	Respiratory insufficiency
		Oral or parenteral antibiotics
		Nebulization of:
		   Mucolytics: dornase alfa
		   Hypertonic saline
		   Antibiotics
		Physiotherapy
		Additional oxygen, NIPPV*
		Lung transplantation

ENT	Nasal polyps Chronic rhinosinusitis	Nasal saline irrigation Topical steroids Antibiotics Endoscopic sinus surgery
Gastrointestinal system	Meconium ileus DIOS* Constipation Gastroesophageal reflux Rectal prolapse	Gastrografin enema, surgery Laxatives, enemas, intestinal lavage PPIs*
Pancreas	Exocrine pancreatic insufficiency Pancreatitis CF-related diabetes	Oral replacement of pancreatic enzymes + PPI Insulin
Hepatobiliary system	Steatosis hepatic Liver cirrhosis Gallstones	UDCA,* liver transplantation UDCA, surgery

Reproductive health	CBAVD in males
	Female subfertility due to several causes
	  (see text)
		MESA, PESA, TESE*
		Assisted reproductive treatment
		  tailored to the cause of
		  subfertility

Growth, maturation	Malabsorption, poor growth
	Pubertal delay
	Osteopenia/osteoporosis
		Vitamin D + vitamin K
		  supplementation, calcium,
		  bisphosphonates

Other	Arthropathia/arthritis Nephrolithiasis Vasculitis Urinary incontinence in women Depression	

* NIPPV = non-invasive positive pressure ventilation; DIOS = distal intestinal obstruction syndrome; PPIs = proton pump inhibitors; UDCA = ursodeoxycholic acid; MESA = microepididymal sperm aspiration; PESA = percutaneous epididymal sperm aspiration; TESE = testicular excisional sperm extraction.

diagnosis, adherence to and access to therapy, and centralization of care. Measurement of the forced expiratory volume (FEV_1) remains the best prognostic predictor. It is the amount of air which can be forcibly expired in 1 second after maximal inspiration. It reflects airway resistance. FEV_1 greater than or equal to 90% predicted is considered normal. Seventy to 89% indicates mild lung disease, 40 to 69% moderate lung disease; less than 40% is a sign of severe lung disease. The annual rate of decline of FEV_1 in CF patients without exacerbations is 1.2%, in CF patients with exacerbations 2.5%.[20]

CF and Pregnancy: Figures

In 1960, the first pregnancy in a patient with CF was reported.[21] The woman died 6 weeks after delivery. The largest study on CF and pregnancy is a nationwide study by Goss[22] describing 680 pregnant patients enrolled in the US Cystic Fibrosis Foundation National Patient Registry between 1985 and 1997 and matching them to non-pregnant control women with CF. Since 2001 the US Cystic Fibrosis Foundation registers 180–220 pregnant women each year.[3] Other nationwide data have come from France,[23] the Netherlands,[2] Israel,[24] Norway and Sweden,[25,26] the UK,[27,28] Canada,[29] and the United States.[30,31] Publications between 1960 and 1991, covering 217 pregnancies in total, were reviewed in 1993 by Kent and Farquharson.[32] Three recent single-centre studies, including a review,[33–35] reported on the outcome of almost 1500 pregnancies in publications thereafter in women who have benefitted from the improvement in prognosis and changed attitude of their medical teams.

Effects of CF on Reproduction

Influence of CF on Fertility

CF has an ill-defined influence on female reproduction. CFTR is present in virtually every part of the human body, including the genital tract. Animal models have shown that it plays a role in ovulation, as well as in fallopian tube and uterine environment. Nevertheless figures on reported (low) fertility should be interpreted with care as not only physical health issues play a role in the decision to try for a pregnancy but also attitudes of CF patients, their family and caregivers towards the broader impact of the disease. While in the past women with CF were believed to have severely impaired fertility, the current conviction is that fertility in women with CF is less compromised thanks to improved health. As to factual data, a population-based cohort study of 1143 CF patients registered with the UK CF Database reported that only 5.7% of women became parents and 0.5% sought fertility treatment.[27] In a Scandinavian study[26] 46 of 61 (75%) women wishing to conceive became pregnant, 34 spontaneously, 7 with intrauterine insemination (IUI) and 5 with *IVF*. A recent British study described 48 pregnancies in patients with CF, 5 conceived via IVF.[34] Miscarriage and ectopic pregnancy rates in these cohorts seemed similar to those in the general population. Boyd et al.[27] reported that women who conceived were less likely to be homozygous for the F508del mutation (OR [odds ratio] 0.48, 95% CI [confidence interval] 0.26–0.89) or to have a poor respiratory health ($FEV_1 < 50\%$, OR 0.56, 95% CI 0.32–0.94).

The particular mechanisms implicated in fertility regulation in women with CF are only starting to emerge. In the past the most likely cause of subfertility was thought to be the thickened cervical mucus. Currently it is clear from human and animal studies that CFTR is implicated in many more processes. Expression of the CFTR in the reproductive tract varies with specific life phases: Significant levels have been demonstrated during the first year of life, decreasing or disappearing thereafter and increasing again after puberty. Expression is highest in the cervix but also is present in endometrium and fallopian tubes.[36] Cervical mucus contains less water and is also less responsive to periovulatory estrogens.

Recent animal studies implicated defective CFTR in altering fallopian tube and uterine fluid excretion and composition, negatively influencing sperm transport and capacitation.[37] These results must however be interpreted with caution as they pertain mostly to in vitro studies.

With menarche being the first hallmark of reproductive life, girls with CF, even those in good clinical condition, have a 2-year delayed menarche as compared to girls without CF (14.9 ± 1.4 years in girls with CF vs. 13.1 ± 1.0 years in controls, $P < 0.001$).[38] Also girls homozygous for the F508del mutation are significantly older at menarche than girls who are heterozygous for this mutation. Finally girls with an abnormal oral glucose tolerance test (oGTT) are significantly older at menarche than girls with a normal oGTT. After menarche, most of these girls establish a regular menstrual pattern, but, in a later case control study, a higher percentage of women with CF than expected from the previous study developed anovulation.[39] CFTR is expressed in the human anterior hypothalamus.[40] In animal studies defective CFTR expression negatively affected aromatase expression and thus estrogen production in ovarian granulosa cells, potentially leading to ovulatory disturbances.[41]

In conclusion, although there are no hard data on subfertility in women with CF, it is realistic to expect that some women with CF may have ovulatory disturbances, unfavourable cervical mucus characteristics, and other impairments in the genital tract and will therefore take recourse to assisted reproduction.

Influence of CF on Pregnancy and Fetus

Recent well-documented series have allowed better-founded advice to be given to women with CF considering pregnancy. Improvement in pregnancy outcome is probably not only an effect of better health care but also reflects better preconception advice for or against pregnancy. Most women with CF in the recent series delivered healthy children. Induced preterm delivery for maternal reasons is the most common complication. CF patients with a pre-pregnancy lung function in the lower range ($FEV_1 < 40$–60%) are at increased risk of delivering prematurely and of giving birth to children with a lower birth weight.[28,33,34] Gestational diabetes develops in over 14% of women with CF.[42] Fifty percent of women delivered via caesarean section, mostly for maternal reasons but also because of breech position associated with earlier delivery. The median birthweight centile was around 32 in the recent UK study.[34] In a Scandinavian study 80% of the babies were breastfed, although in all cases only for 3 months.[25] Breast milk of CF patients contains the appropriate nutrients.[43]

Influence of Pregnancy on Disease Progression, Morbidity and Survival of the CF Patient

Several studies in pregnant CF patients did not show an aggravating effect of pregnancy on lung function decline in pregnant CF patients as compared to matched non-pregnant CF patients.[28,33,34] Women in a stable pulmonary and nutritional condition receiving good medical care usually are considered at low risk for disease deterioration. Better patient compliance and intensified medical supervision might have a beneficial influence. Pre-pregnancy FEV_1 and body mass index (BMI) are good predictors for both maternal and child outcome. The average weight gain of a patient with CF in a Scandinavian series[25] was 10 kg (19% increase of body weight) which is normal.

Fifty percent of women, all with pancreatic insufficiency, needed nutritional supplements either via a nasogastric tube or parenterally. The need for intravenous antibiotics was doubled during pregnancy as compared to the pre- or post-pregnancy period. Lung function did not deteriorate. Four of 23 women developed gestational diabetes, in concordance with data from other studies.[29,30] A matched control study covering 216 CF patients from the US Registry, pregnant between 1995 and 2003, showed that pregnant CF patients suffered from bacterial respiratory infections more frequently, had higher hospitalization rates and needed more antibiotic courses. Also the prevalence of diabetes more than doubled. Only in about half of the cases diabetes resolved after pregnancy.[30]

Maternal survival has been studied in the US registry as well. There were 680 CF patients, who became pregnant between 1985 and 1997, followed on the long term. Women who became pregnant did not have a significantly shortened survival as compared to their matched controls. Post-delivery survival after 10 years was about 80% in CF patients with a good ($FEV_1 > 80\%$) pre-pregnancy lung function but only 60% in those with a poor ($FEV_1 < 40\%$) pre-pregnancy lung function.[44] The median maternal survival in a study from the UK covering 72 pregnancies was 11.9 years after the birth of the first child. In women delivering preterm this median survival was 7.6 years.[28] In a more recent series 4 of 9 patients with an FEV_1 40–50% died between 2 and 8 years after delivery, whereas 3 of 5 with an $FEV_1 < 40\%$ died within 18 months after delivery.[34] Factors associated with a bad prognosis where pregnancy is contraindicated are listed in Table 1.3.[45-48] Respiratory complications have the greatest impact on survival.

Not only pregnancy but also motherhood and its demands could have a long-term worsening effect on (perceived) health. This was elegantly studied by Schechter et al.,[49] who questioned 119 CF mothers and 1190 matched controls a median range of 6 years after pregnancy. Pregnancy and motherhood came with more illness-related visits, pulmonary exacerbations and a decrease in some aspects of quality of life probably reflecting the effect of motherhood on disease management (Figure 1.2).

The most difficult part of pre-pregnancy counselling is to confront both partners with the many aspects of deteriorating health, need for transplantation, parenthood in

TABLE 1.3

Predictors of Poor Prognosis in CF

Absolute Contraindications for Pregnancy
$FEV_1 < 30\%$ predicted or rapid decline in FEV_1
Hypoxia, hypercarbia
Pulmonary hypertension
Severe liver disease with portal hypertension

Relative Contraindications for Pregnancy
Poor nutritional state: hypoalbuminemia, wasting
 Poor weight for height (BMI < 18 kg/m^2)
Frequent respiratory infections
Massive hemoptysis
Recurrent pneumothorax
Colonization by *Burkholderia cepacia* strains

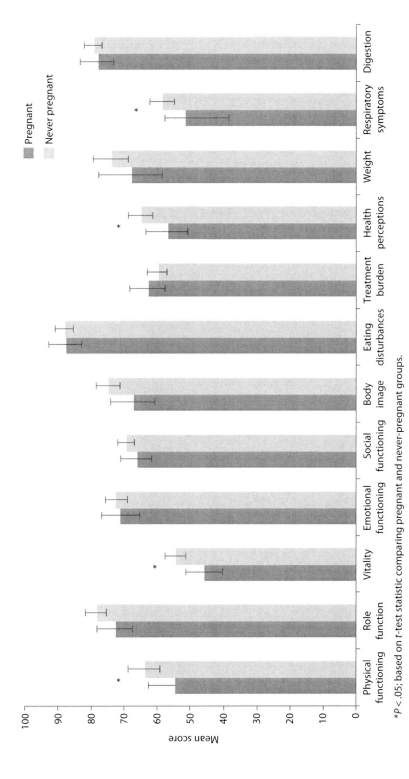

FIGURE 1.2 Scores on the Cystic Fibrosis Questionnaire–Revised during the endpoint period 2004 to 2005. Comparison of women who had reported a pregnancy to those who had not. (From Schechter MS, Quittner AL, Konstan MW, et al. Ann Am Thorac Soc 2013;10:213–9. With permission of the publisher and the first author.)

*$P < .05$; based on t-test statistic comparing pregnant and never-pregnant groups.

these situations, and eventually death with a young child to leave behind. In general one can say that 1 in 5 children will be raised without a mother at the age of 10 years. In patients with unfavourable parameters (FEV_1 below 40% or diabetes) this will be the case for 2 in 5 children.[22] This means that long-term issues such as the support of the husband and family should be discussed openly and timely.

Pregnancy after Lung Transplantation

In general the 2-year survival of a CF patient with an $FEV_1 \leq 30\%$, is about 50%.[45] When a patient reaches this critical figure, he or she has to consider the possibility of lung transplantation. After lung transplantation CF patients have a median survival of 5.5 years in most transplantation centres. Conditional on survival of at least 1 year, overall median survival was 7.8 years.[50] In some transplantation centres median survival was more than 10 years.[51] Individual predictions of survival are difficult to make. There are few data on pregnancies after lung transplantation in CF patients. Gyi et al.[52] described ten cases from the UK. Four mothers showed rejection during pregnancy. One of them already had symptoms before pregnancy, however. All four died of chronic rejection within 38 months after delivery. The other six women were stable 1–6 years after delivery. As to the fetal outcome, one pregnancy was terminated, the other nine ended with live birth, and although some infants were premature, all did well at follow-up. Lung transplantation is generally considered as a contraindication for pregnancy, and this is certainly the case in patients showing episodes of rejection and in patients with obliterative bronchiolitis. A minimum interval of 1 year after transplantation is to be recommended to allow assessment of graft function. Case-by-case advice should be given. Co-morbidity and medication have to be taken into account as well.

Decision Making

More than half of the women interviewed in a Scandinavian study[26] did not pursue pregnancy. Reasons to refrain from pregnancy are difficulties in finding a partner, reluctance towards medical interventions, being physically not fit enough, lack of excess energy to raise a child, fear of complications, uncertainty about the future, reduced life expectancy, and not wishing to transmit disease or carriership. In rare cases there has been a request for surrogate motherhood. CF patients usually need 2–4 hours a day for airway cleaning, nebulization, administration of medication (local and systemic) and physiotherapy. On one hand, having a child may give a new purpose to life and enhance motivation to undertake these daily tasks; on the other hand, care of the newborn may entail a time constraint prohibiting adequate self-care. Also, young children increase the infectious load with a family unit.

A second issue is the health and happiness of the child. The child will have a parent with a progressive chronic disease and experience the restrictions this entails for family life and activities. The child might become a caregiver at a young age. He or she eventually will lose a parent at a young age. On the other hand the child will realise that being healthy is not to be taken for granted. Finally the child is by definition a carrier of one CF mutation and in due time will have to inform a potential partner.

A beautiful study of decision-making, containing many valuable cross references,[53] summarized relevant issues as expressed in semi-structured interviews by 12 women with CF who were otherwise well as characterized by health status, QOL (quality of life) and psychological well-being. Four core categories emerged, each containing a number of subcategories (Figure 1.3). There were issues that also apply to women without a chronic disease, such as "I want to be normal" and the questions "Is wanting a child a selfish act?" "What is the right timing?" "Am I going to be a good parent?" "Is my relationship strong enough to cope with the unpredictable demands of a child?" And there were issues related with having CF: "Is my life going to be shortened by pregnancy and parenthood?" "What will be the impact of me being sick or dying early on my child?" Women expressed the importance of early information (before embarking into a relationship) and of the opinion of the medical team. Overall it appeared "that women with CF make a dynamic decision about pregnancy which is subject to many different factors at different points in time". None of the 12 participants had considered assisted reproduction.

The knowledge of the partner of a CF patient should be ascertained, and one must make sure that the partner is involved in all steps of decision-making. The social network and family support should be assessed so that in case of maternal deterioration or early demise, care for the child is guaranteed.

Preparing for Pregnancy

A thorough pre-pregnancy assessment and multidisciplinary consultation should precede any pregnancy in a woman with CF. The assessment should include pulmonary function (FEV), sputum cultures, BMI, hemoglobin A1c, oGTT, adaptation of medication and diet, and carrier testing of the partner if so wished. The consultation team includes the pulmonologist, endocrinologist, geneticist, reproductive medicine physician, obstetrician, anaesthesiologist and counsellor. In some cases a medical ethical team may have to be consulted, especially if the couple requests assisted reproductive techniques and there is doubt about the maternal prognosis.

Pregnancy should be discouraged in cases with an $FEV_1 \leq 30\%$, pulmonary arterial hypertension, hypercarbia, and severe liver disease with portal hypertension (Table 1.3). A BMI below 20 kg/m^2 and a FEV_1 below 60% of predicted are relative contraindications because they are associated with a significant increase of the risk for (iatrogenic) pre-term delivery. In severe pancreatic dysfunction, reaching an adequate weight gain during pregnancy will be difficult.

In women who do not want to conceive, contraception is indicated, as women with CF are usually fertile. Although pharmacokinetic studies have shown adequate concentrations of estradiol in 3 CF patients receiving 50 μg ethinylestradiol orally and no systemic antibiotics,[52,54] multiple drug interactions, malabsorption, diarrhoea and liver disease with disturbed enterohepatic circulation may diminish the bioavailability of oral contraceptives sometimes but not always heralded by breakthrough bleeding. An inventory among 55 women with CF in Australia (median age 22 years) revealed the rather disturbing fact that a majority of them believed that their fertility

IVF in the Medically Complicated Patient

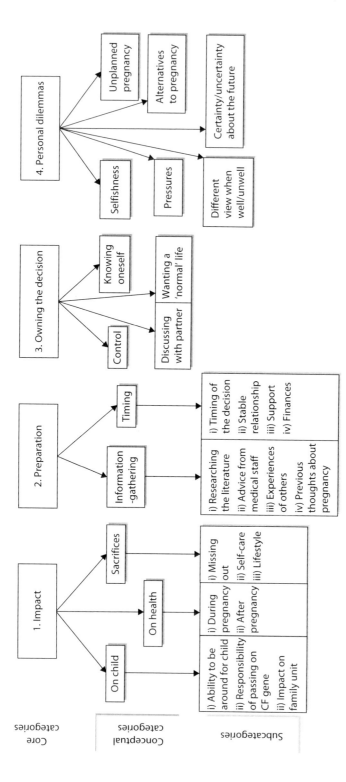

FIGURE 1.3 Diagrammatic representation of factors in decision-making. (From Simcox AM, Hewison J, Duff AJ, Morton AM, Conway SP. Br J Health Psychol 2009;14:323–42. With permission of the publisher.)

was reduced and therefore did not use contraception. Furthermore the awareness of the potential adverse effects of pregnancy on disease and vice versa was low.[55,56]

It is strongly recommended that the partner be tested for CF mutations as well. When screening for the most common 35 mutations in a North European partner, if none is detected, the resultant risk of CF in the offspring is estimated to be 1 in 1500. Reproductive choices when the partner is also a carrier are to accept the 50% risk of a child with CF, to have prenatal diagnosis followed by eventual termination of pregnancy, to refrain from having children, to use donor gametes, and finally to use *in vitro* fertilization (IVF) in combination with pre-implantation genetic diagnosis (PGD). CF was the first autosomal monogenic disorder for which PGD became available.[57] PGD in affected females has been described in cases of compound heterozygosity with less-severe mutations such as a class V mutation combined with F508del.[58,59] In such cases the difficult ethical question can arise whether or not to transfer an embryo with a classic and a less-severe mutation. Such individual requests require careful evaluation.

If unprotected intercourse does not lead to a pregnancy within 6 months we advise cycle evaluation, and after 12 months of unprotected intercourse additional assessment of the risk of tubal non-patency and semen analysis. When determining a chlamydial antibody titer, cross reactions with antibodies against *Chlamydia pneumonia* should be excluded before proceeding to invasive tubal patency tests. A schematic recommendation for fertility assessment and treatment is presented in Figure 1.4.

Assisted Reproduction in Women with CF

Little is known about ART in women with CF. In a case series of five women, three conceived after IUI and two after IVF.[60] Two women were homozygous for F508del, two were compound heterozygous with F508del involved, one was compound heterozygous for other mutations. With so little data to rely on, advice on how to conduct ART in women with CF is by nature authority based. Common sense leads to the notion that avoiding multiple pregnancy is crucial. The CF patient is unable to cope with the increased nutritional, mechanical and ventilatory demands of a multiple pregnancy. This implies prudent ovarian stimulation and strict cancellation criteria in case of ovulation induction or ovarian hyperstimulation, IUI in a natural cycle, and single-embryo transfer at IVF. Despite its possible negative effect on cervical mucus, clomiphene citrate, if necessary combined with IUI, is the first drug of choice for ovulation induction because of its low risk of multiple pregnancy. In patients with recurrent pulmonary infections it might be prudent not to schedule IVF treatment in the cold and wet season. As many as 24% of women with CF report recurrent vulvovaginal candidiasis due to the use of antibiotics. Treatment is recommended among other reasons to prevent colonization of the oocyte and embryo cultures in the laboratory. Oral fluconazol has been reported to be safe also during early pregnancy.[61]

Management during Early Pregnancy

If the partner is a carrier and all mutations are known, prenatal diagnosis via direct mutation analysis is possible in the first trimester in chorionic villi and in the second trimester in amniotic fluid. In view of the 50% risk of an affected child, early

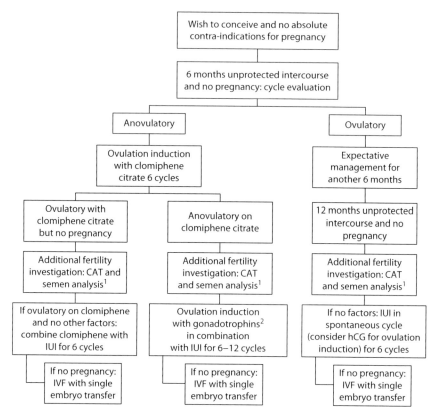

FIGURE 1.4 Flowchart of management in case of wish to conceive. 1, if CAT (computerized axial tomography) and/or semen analysis abnormal, follow usual fertility protocols; 2, apply gradual low-dose step-up schedule and strict cancellation criteria or consider proceeding to IVF directly.

diagnosis will be preferred by most couples. In the case that not all three relevant mutations are known, linkage studies in chorionic villi can enable prenatal diagnosis provided the diagnosis of CF and paternity are certain and provided living affected and non-affected family members are available and willing to cooperate in giving blood samples. It is strongly recommended to set up such a linkage study before an actual pregnancy. In case the paternal mutation differs from the maternal mutations, the paternal mutation can be identified in maternal plasma, hence avoiding invasive prenatal diagnosis.[62–64] This technology is however not yet routinely available.

In case of multiple pregnancy serious thought should be given to selective feticide in order to achieve a singleton pregnancy.

Any physician caring for a woman with CF who wishes to become pregnant or is pregnant already will tremendously benefit from the recently published guidelines, based on expert consensus, for the management of pregnancy in women with cystic fibrosis.[65] Pregnancy care in specialized CF centres focuses on adapting medication, optimising lung function and nutritional status, early diagnosis of gestational diabetes, and adapting physiotherapy according to the stage and the requirements of pregnancy.

The CF nurse is, as before, the liaison officer coordinating the care in such a way that it is maximally time effective for the patient. The number of physicians involved in the care will increase during pregnancy and now also include an obstetrician, an obstetric anaesthesiologist and a clinical geneticist.

Most medications used to treat CF are safe for use in pregnancy (Table 1.4). Prophylactic treatment does not have to be altered. Multi-drug-resistant organisms may however force use of agents with less-extensive pregnancy data. Pulmonary exacerbations and infections should be treated aggressively because of their associated risk of premature delivery. Common pathogens in respiratory tract infections in adult CF patients are *Pseudomonas aeruginosa*, *Staphylococcus aureus* and sometimes *Haemophilus influenzae*. Pulmonary function, oxygen saturation, sputum cultures and measurement of weight should be done at intervals of at least 4 weeks. A regular assessment of lung function and nutrition is essential.

Pregnancy requires an additional 300 kcal per day. Failure to gain weight is associated with an increased rate of premature delivery, and therefore it is important to install nasogastric tube or gastrostomy feeding or rarely parenteral feeding when nutritional problems become apparent. Additional essential fatty acids, minerals, fat-soluble vitamins (A, D and K), iron and folic acid in the appropriate dosages for pregnancy may be required because of resorption disturbances. Iron resorption can be optimised by increasing the intake of vitamin C. Vitamin A should not be given in dosages exceeding

TABLE 1.4

Safety during Pregnancy of Antibiotics Commonly Used in CF Patients

Antibiotics	Category	Comment
Penicillins	A-B1	Safe to use in pregnancy
Azithromycin	B1	Safe
Tetracycline	D	Avoid second and third trimester
Ciprofloxacin Fluoroquininolones	B3	Avoid; in animal testing fetal cartilage defects
Trimethoprim/ Sulfamethoxazole	C	Avoid first and third trimester
Aminoglycosides	D	Inhaled tobramycin in low dose is not toxic Tobramycin intravenous not in first trimester In second and third trimester once-daily dosing and with drug level monitoring
Vancomycin	B2	Unknown; no evidence of fetal damage
Imepenem	B3	Avoid in pregnancy
Colistin	B2	Inhalation is safe; avoid intravenous usage in pregnancy

Notes: A. Drugs have been used widely in pregnancy and are assumed to be safe for the fetus.

B. Drugs not known to cause harm to the human fetus but with insufficient experience to consider them safe.

B1. Drugs that have been demonstrated to cause no harm in animal studies.

B2. Drugs with insufficient animal data.

B3. Drugs that have been demonstrated to harm the fetus in animal studies.

C. Drugs that could theoretically cause harm to the fetus by their pharmacological actions.

D. Drugs known or believed to cause harm to the fetus.

10,000 IU per day. Common CF gastrointestinal problems such as reflux, dyspepsia, vomiting, obstipation may be aggravated during pregnancy and should be tackled preventively. Some women have problems of cholestasis and the associated pruritus that can be excruciating. Ursodeoxycholic acid can be beneficial here. Bile acid levels above 100μmol/L indicate severe cholestasis and are associated with an increased risk of spontaneous preterm birth, meconium stained amniotic fluid and perinatal death. Patients with diabetes should be monitored according to a diabetes protocol. Those who have not developed diabetes should undergo screening for gestational diabetes at 24 weeks. Glucose levels should be monitored during episodes of infection and during delivery.

Reflection

Care for women with CF wishing to conceive benefits from a multidisciplinary approach where the team members have interest in and knowledge about CF and interact well. In view of the rarity of the condition the care should be done in or in close collaboration with a CF centre. Continuity of care is important. With earlier diagnosis and better treatment of CF from childhood on, more women will receive a positive answer to their question whether pregnancy and parenthood are attainable goals.

WEBSITES

www.cfww.org
www.cysticfibrosismedicine.com
http://www.genet.sickkids.on.ca/cftr/app
http://www.ncfs

REFERENCES

1. Dodge JA, Lewis PA, Stanton M, Wilsher J. Cystic fibrosis mortality and survival in the UK: 1947–2003. *Eur Resp J* 2007;29:522–6.
2. Slieker MG, Uiterwaal CS, Sinaasappel M, Heijerman HG, van der Laag J, van der Ent CK. Birth prevalence and survival in cystic fibrosis: a national cohort study in the Netherlands. *Chest* 2005;128:2309–15.
3. Cystic Fibrosis Foundation Patient Registry 2011 Annual Report. Bethesda, MD, 2012:1–30.
4. Sims EJ, Clark A, McCormick J, et al. Cystic fibrosis diagnosed after 2 months of age leads to worse outcomes and requires more therapy. *Pediatrics* 2007;119:19–28.
5. Dijk FN, McKay K, Barzi F, Gaskin KJ, Fitzgerald DA. Improved survival in cystic fibrosis patients diagnosed by newborn screening compared to a historical cohort from the same centre. *Arch Dis Child* 2011;96:1118–23.
6. Farrell PM. The prevalence of cystic fibrosis in the European Union. *J Cyst Fibros* 2008;7:450–3.
7. Strausbaugh SD, Davis PB. Cystic fibrosis: a review of epidemiology and pathobiology. *Clin Chest Med* 2007;28:279–88.
8. Scotet V, Audrezet MP, Roussey M, et al. Impact of public health strategies on the birth prevalence of cystic fibrosis in Brittany, France. *Hum Genet* 2003;113:280–5.

9. Hale JE, Parad RB, Comeau AM. Newborn screening showing decreasing incidence of cystic fibrosis. *N Engl J Med* 2008;358:973–4.
10. Kerem B, Rommens JM, Buchanan JA, et al. Identification of the cystic fibrosis gene: genetic analysis. *Science* 1989;245:1073–80.
11. Riordan JR, Rommens JM, Kerem B, et al. Identification of the cystic fibrosis gene: cloning and characterization of complementary DNA. *Science* 1989;245:1066–73.
12. Rommens JM, Iannuzzi MC, Kerem B, et al. Identification of the cystic fibrosis gene: chromosome walking and jumping. *Science* 1989;245:1059–65.
13. Kerem E. Pharmacological induction of CFTR function in patients with cystic fibrosis: mutation-specific therapy. *Pediatr Pulmonol* 2005;40:183–96.
14. Amaral MD, Kunzelmann K. Molecular targeting of CFTR as a therapeutic approach to cystic fibrosis. *Trends Pharmacol Sci* 2007;28:334–41.
15. Ameen N, Silvis M, Bradbury NA. Endocytic trafficking of CFTR in health and disease. *J Cyst Fibros* 2007;6:1–14.
16. Zeitlin PL. Novel pharmacologic therapies for cystic fibrosis. *J Clin Invest* 1999;103:447–52.
17. Ratjen F. New pulmonary therapies for cystic fibrosis. *Curr Opin Pulm Med* 2007;13:541–6.
18. McKone EF, Emerson SS, Edwards KL, Aitken ML. Effect of genotype on phenotype and mortality in cystic fibrosis: a retrospective cohort study. *Lancet* 2003;361:1671–6.
19. Knowles MR, Drumm M. The influence of genetics on cystic fibrosis phenotypes. *Cold Spring Harb Perspect Med* 2012;2:a009548.
20. Waters V, Stanojevic S, Atenafu EG, et al. Effect of pulmonary exacerbations on long-term lung function decline in cystic fibrosis. *Eur Resp J* 2012;40:61–6.
21. Siegel B, Siegel S. Pregnancy and delivery in a patient with cystic fibrosis of the pancreas. *Obstet Gynecol* 1960;16:438–40.
22. Goss CH, Rubenfeld GD, Otto K, Aitken ML. The effect of pregnancy on survival in women with cystic fibrosis. *Chest* 2003;124:1460–8.
23. Gillet D, de Braekeleer M, Bellis G, Durieu I. Cystic fibrosis and pregnancy. Report from French data (1980–1999). *BJOG* 2002;109:912–8.
24. Barak A, Dulitzki M, Efrati O, et al. Pregnancies and outcome in women with cystic fibrosis. *Isr Med Assoc J* 2005;7:95–8.
25. Odegaard I, Stray-Pedersen B, Hallberg K, Haanaes OC, Storrosten OT, Johannesson M. Maternal and fetal morbidity in pregnancies of Norwegian and Swedish women with cystic fibrosis. *Acta Obstet Gynecol Scand* 2002;81:698–705.
26. Odegaard I, Stray-Pedersen B, Hallberg K, Haanaes OC, Storrosten OT, Johannesson M. Prevalence and outcome of pregnancies in Norwegian and Swedish women with cystic fibrosis. *Acta Obstet Gynecol Scand* 2002;81:693–7.
27. Boyd JM, Mehta A, Murphy DJ. Fertility and pregnancy outcomes in men and women with cystic fibrosis in the United Kingdom. *Hum Reprod* 2004;19:2238–43.
28. Edenborough FP, Mackenzie WE, Stableforth DE. The outcome of 72 pregnancies in 55 women with cystic fibrosis in the United Kingdom 1977–1996. *BJOG* 2000;107:254–61.
29. Gilljam M, Antoniou M, Shin J, Dupuis A, Corey M, Tullis DE. Pregnancy in cystic fibrosis. Fetal and maternal outcome. *Chest* 2000;118:85–91.
30. McMullen AH, Pasta DJ, Frederick PD, et al. Impact of pregnancy on women with cystic fibrosis. *Chest* 2006;129:706–11.
31. Cheng EY, Goss CH, McKone EF, et al. Aggressive prenatal care results in successful fetal outcomes in CF women. *J Cyst Fibros* 2006;5:85–91.

32. Kent NE, Farquharson DF. Cystic fibrosis in pregnancy. *CMAJ* 1993;149:809–13.
33. Lau EM, Barnes DJ, Moriarty C, et al. Pregnancy outcomes in the current era of cystic fibrosis care: a 15-year experience. *Aust N Z J Obstet Gynaecol* 2011;51:220–4.
34. Thorpe-Beeston JG, Madge S, Gyi K, Hodson M, Bilton D. The outcome of pregnancies in women with cystic fibrosis – single centre experience 1998–2011. *BJOG* 2013;120:354–61.
35. Burden C, Ion R, Chung Y, Henry A, Downey DG, Trinder J. Current pregnancy outcomes in women with cystic fibrosis. *Eur J Obstet Gynecol Reprod Biol* 2012;164:142–5.
36. Tizzano EF, Silver MM, Chitayat D, et al. Differential cellular expression of cystic fibrosis transmembrane regulator in human reproductive tissues. *Am J Pathol* 1994;144:906–14.
37. Hodges CA, Palmert MR, Drumm ML. Infertility in females with cystic fibrosis is multifactorial: evidence from mouse models. *Endocrinology* 2008;149:2790–7.
38. Johannesson M, Gottlieb C, Hjelte L. Delayed puberty in girls with cystic fibrosis despite good clinical status. *Pediatrics* 1997;99:29–34.
39. Johannesson M, Landgren BM, Csemiczky G, Hjelte L, Gottlieb C. Female patients with cystic fibrosis suffer from reproductive endocrinological disorders despite good clinical status. *Hum Reprod* 1998;13:2092–7.
40. Mulberg AE WR, Altschuler SM, Hyde TM. Cystic fibrosis transmembrane conductance regulator expression in human hypothalamus. *NeuroReport* 1998;9:141–4.
41. Chen H, Guo JH, Lu YC, et al. Impaired CFTR-dependent amplification of FSH-stimulated estrogen production in cystic fibrosis and PCOS. *J Clin Endocrinol Metab* 2012;97:923–32.
42. Gilljam M. Pregnancy in cystic fibrosis. Fetal and maternal outcome. *Chest* 2000;118:85.
43. Johannesson M. Effects of pregnancy on health: certain aspects of importance for women with cystic fibrosis. *J Cyst Fibros* 2002;1:9–12.
44. Goss CH. The effect of pregnancy on survival in women with cystic fibrosis. *Chest* 2003;124:1460–8.
45. Kerem E, Reisman J, Corey M, Canny GJ, Levison H. Prediction of mortality in patients with cystic fibrosis. *N Engl J Med* 1992;326:1187–91.
46. Mayer-Hamblett N, Rosenfeld M, Emerson J, Goss CH, Aitken ML. Developing cystic fibrosis lung transplant referral criteria using predictors of 2-year mortality. *Am J Respir Crit Care Med* 2002;166:1550–5.
47. Johnson C, Butler SM, Konstan MW, Morgan W, Wohl ME. Factors influencing outcomes in cystic fibrosis: a center-based analysis. *Chest* 2003;123:20–7.
48. Courtney JM, Bradley J, McCaughan J, et al. Predictors of mortality in adults with cystic fibrosis. *Pediatric Pulmonol* 2007;42:525–32.
49. Schechter MS, Quittner AL, Konstan MW, et al. Long-term effects of pregnancy and motherhood on disease outcomes of women with cystic fibrosis. *Ann Am Thorac Soc* 2013;10:213–9.
50. Christie JD, Edwards LB, Kucheryavaya AY, et al. The Registry of the International Society for Heart and Lung Transplantation: twenty-eighth adult lung and heart-lung transplant report – 2011. *J Heart Lung Transplant* 2011;30:1104–22.
51. Meachery G, De Soyza A, Nicholson A, et al. Outcomes of lung transplantation for cystic fibrosis in a large UK cohort. *Thorax* 2008;63:725–31.
52. Gyi KM, Hodson ME, Yacoub MY. Pregnancy in cystic fibrosis lung transplant recipients: case series and review. *J Cyst Fibros* 2006;5:171–5.
53. Simcox AM, Hewison J, Duff AJ, Morton AM, Conway SP. Decision-making about pregnancy for women with cystic fibrosis. *Br J Health Psychol* 2009;14:323–42.

54. Stead RJ, Grimmer SF, Rogers SM, et al. Pharmacokinetics of contraceptive steroids in patients with cystic fibrosis. *Thorax* 1987;42:59–64.
55. Sawyer SM PP, Bowes G. Reproductive health in young women with cystic fibrosis: knowledge, behavior and attitudes. *J Adolesc Health* 1995;17:46–50.
56. Sawyer SM. Reproductive health in young people with cystic fibrosis. *Curr Opin Pediatr* 1995;7:376–80.
57. Handyside AH, Lesko JG, Tarin JJ, Winston RM, Hughes MR. Birth of a normal girl after *in vitro* fertilization and preimplantation diagnostic testing for cystic fibrosis. *N Engl J Med* 1992;327:905–9.
58. Keymolen K, Goossens V, De Rycke M, et al. Clinical outcome of preimplantation genetic diagnosis for cystic fibrosis: the Brussels' experience. *Eur J Hum Genet* 2007;15:752–8.
59. Rechitsky S, Verlinsky O, Kuliev A. PGD for cystic fibrosis patients and couples at risk of an additional genetic disorder combined with 24-chromosome aneuploidy testing. *Reprod Biomed Online* 2013;26:420–30.
60. Epelboin S, Hubert D, Patrat C, et al. Management of assisted reproductive technologies in women with cystic fibrosis. *Fertil Steril* 2001;76:1280–1.
61. Molgaard-Nielsen D, Pasternak B, Hviid A. Use of oral fluconazole during pregnancy and the risk of birth defects. *N Engl J Med* 2013;369:830–9.
62. Gonzalez-Gonzalez MC, Garcia-Hoyos M, Trujillo MJ, et al. Prenatal detection of a cystic fibrosis mutation in fetal DNA from maternal plasma. *Prenat Diagn* 2002;22:946–8.
63. Norbury G, Norbury CJ. Non-invasive prenatal diagnosis of single gene disorders: how close are we? *Semin Fetal Neonatal Med* 2008;13:76–83.
64. Bustamante-Aragones A, Gallego-Merlo J, Trujillo-Tiebas MJ, et al. New strategy for the prenatal detection/exclusion of paternal cystic fibrosis mutations in maternal plasma. *J Cyst Fibros* 2008;7:505–10.
65. Edenborough FP, Borgo G, Knoop C, Lannefors L, et al. Guidelines for the management of pregnancy in women with cystic fibrosis. *J Cyst Fibros* 2008;7:S2–S32.

2

The Patient at Risk from Thrombosis

NS Macklon

CONTENTS

Introduction

The clinical association between venous thromboembolism (VTE) and in vitro fertilization (IVF) arises primarily within the context of ovarian hyperstimulation syndrome (OHSS), in which thromboembolic complications may have fatal consequences. Occasionally patients presenting for IVF treatment may have a previous history of VTE or be considered to be at increased risk of developing thromboembolic complications as a result of undergoing IVF treatment. The incidence of VTE following IVF treatment is uncertain, as recent studies have reported varying data ranging from no increased incidence compared to that in age-matched populations[1] to 10-fold increase with the background population. When VTEs occurring in pregnancy are included, the incidence rises to 2.6 per 1000, compared with 0.97 per 1000 in spontaneously conceived pregnancies.[2]

Given the thrombophilic nature of ovarian stimulation and the potentially catastrophic effects of VTE, it is important to identify women at increased potential risk of this complication, so as to provide appropriate counselling and allow preventive steps to be taken where necessary. While fortunately rare in this patient group, venous thrombosis is a potentially serious disorder, which may often lead to post-thrombotic syndrome causing chronic morbidity. In one study of long-term complications, 74% of women with upper-extremity deep venous thrombosis (DVT) had residual disability up to 6 years later in the form of persistent discomfort, exercise-induced cramp, cold hands and weakness.[3] Since women undergoing IVF are on the whole young and active, this may afflict their lives for many years. In this chapter, the mechanisms thought to increase the risk of thrombogenesis during IVF treatment are reviewed, strategies for identifying the at-risk patient are discussed, and management options aimed at reducing the risk are summarised.

The Impact of IVF on the Risk of Thromboembolic Disease

The pathogenesis of venous thrombosis is complex and not completely understood. The classic triad of predisposing mechanisms described by Virchow – hypercoagulability, venous stasis and vascular damage – is still of value in understanding circumstances that may lead to DVT in the context of IVF. Ovarian stimulation results in a hyperestrogenic state, which has been associated with hypercoagulability and increased risk of DVT following oral contraceptive pill use and pregnancy. Evidence for estrogens as causes of thrombosis is provided by the reduction in the incidence of DVT associated with lower doses of estrogens in oral contraceptive pills. The supraphysiological levels of estrogens that arise during ovarian stimulation for IVF would therefore appear to cause an increase in the risk of VTE. A recent study indicated that thrombin generation increased after ovarian stimulation, but this was in comparison with the down-regulated state, which does not represent a physiological control. A number of studies have shown changes from baseline in coagulation parameters during IVF treatment to be modest.[4–6] Indeed, during IVF treatment, the action of coagulation factors seems to be associated less with the level of serum estradiol concentrations (which may reach levels ten times higher than in physiological cycles but remain below those occurring in pregnancy) than with the biochemical changes that occur after the triggering of final oocyte maturation with human chorionic gonadotropin (hCG). The predominant contribution of hCG rather than estradiol to the aetiology of VTE after ovarian stimulation is supported by the clinical observation that frozen thaw cycles (when estrogens but not hCG are administered) are not associated with an increased risk compared to natural conceptions.[2]

Taken together, these data suggest that hyperestrogenism related to ovarian stimulation is not associated with the coagulation abnormalities observed with high estrogen content oral contraceptives and therefore does not significantly increase the potential for thrombus formation. During down-regulation and luteal support, the changes in plasma levels of anticoagulant proteins are virtually negligible. The only coagulation parameter that may change considerably during IVF treatment is the activated protein C (APC) resistance.

In its activated form, protein C plays a central role in fibrinolysis. During ovarian stimulation, levels of APC actually appear to increase in association with rising estradiol levels. At the same time, factor VIII and protein S levels are diminished. This slight increase in APC associated with raised estradiol levels might be considered as a protective mechanism against thrombosis during periods of estrogen excess. Indeed, patients resistant to APC have been shown to be at greater risk of thrombosis during ovarian stimulation.

The possibility that ovarian stimulation for IVF treatment increases susceptibility to thrombosis by inducing APC resistance has been suggested. Most of the studies that failed to show such an association employed an APC resistance test that quantifies the effect of APC on the intrinsic coagulation pathway. This pathway is much less sensitive to changes in sex steroids than the tissue factor-based extrinsic coagulation pathway. The extrinsic pathway is initiated by the release of tissue factor, which is released after tissue damage, and stimulated monocytes. The tissue-factor-based APC resistance test used in investigations of the effect of oral contraceptive pills is sensitive to changes in estrogens and does reveal changes during hyperstimulation. In a study in which the effect of ovarian stimulation on the extrinsic pathway was measured, APC sensitivity ratios (APCsr) increased slightly at down-regulation, increased more strongly during hyperstimulation and remained high during the luteal phase. The plasma levels of anticoagulant proteins, protein C and protein S, did not change significantly.[7] However, since thrombin formation is unchanged during ovarian stimulation, increases in tissue plasminogen activator (TPA) are unlikely to be a major concern.

Increases in blood viscosity associated with an increase in haemoglobin (Hb) or haematocrit (hct) (otherwise measured as packed cell volume, PCV) are associated with a greater risk of thrombosis. In this situation, blood flow becomes slow and platelets and neutrophils in the blood circulation adhere easily to the vascular wall, resulting in contact activation of the blood coagulation cascade system. However, studies have indicated that activation of the coagulation system occurs before haemoconcentration can be clinically recognized, a finding inconsistent with the concept that haemoconcentration during IVF is the principal trigger of the coagulation cascade.

Increases in parameters of haemoconcentration have been reported to occur during the period of down-regulation with gonadotropin-releasing hormone (GnRH) agonists prior to commencing ovarian stimulation.[7]

During stimulation, these variables were observed to return to baseline, and in the luteal phase they dropped to values below baseline. The changes in haematocrit were relatively minor.

Given the modest effects of IVF on haemoglobin, haematocrit, platelets and the plasma levels of the proteins involved in the protein C pathway, it seems reasonable to conclude that ovarian stimulation itself (prior to the administration of hCG to trigger final oocyte maturation) induces only marginal changes in haemostatic parameters. In contrast, the period following hCG administration reveals clinically significant alterations in the coagulation and fibrinolytic systems. The changes in these factors before and after hCG administration are summarised in Table 2.1.

Following hCG administration, fibrinogen and factors II, V, VII, VIII and IX are elevated.[4] In one study, activation of the coagulation cascade system was observed to occur within 2 days after hCG, reaching a maximum approximately 8 days following hCG administration.[8] Activation of these systems was observed to continue for more than 3 weeks when pregnancy was established.[8]

Fibrinolysis also increases after hCG administration. However, the fibrinolytic phenomena only occur several days after the thrombotic phenomena have appeared, consistent with a prothrombotic state in the early luteal phase.

Ovarian Hyperstimulation Syndrome

Severe forms of thrombosis following ovarian stimulation for IVF have been reported in women with concomitant signs of OHSS.[8,9] In a recent Swedish cohort study of almost 1 million deliveries the 6% to 7% of IVF pregnancies that were complicated

TABLE 2.1

Overview of Effects of Ovarian Stimulation on Haemostatic
Parameters Compared with Baseline Levels and Data from
Non-Stimulated Cycles

Parameter		**Pre-hCG**	**Post-hCG**
Whole-blood parameters	Haemoglobin	=	↓
	Haematocrit	=	↓
	Platelet count	↓	=
Coagulation inhibitors	Antithrombin	↓	↓/=
	Protein S total	↓	↓/=
	Protein S free	=	=
	Protein C activity	=	↓/=
	Protein C antigen	=	=
	Protein C inhibitor	=	=
	APCsr	↑/=	↑/=
Measures of haemostasis	PT	↑	↓
	APTT	=	↓/=
Clotting factors	Factor I (fibrinogen)	=	↑/=
	Factor II (prothrombin)	=	↑
	Factor V	=	↑
	Factor VII	=	↑
	Factor VIII	=	↑/=
	Factor IX	=	↑
	Factor X	=	=

Source: Data derived from Lox C, Canez M, DeLeon F, et al. Fertil Steril 1995;
63: 566–70; Curvers J, Nap AW, Thomassen MC, et al. Br J Haematol
2001; 115: 400–7; Kodama H, Fukuda J, Karube H, Matsui T, et al.
Fertil Steril 1996; 66: 417–24.

Note: APCsr, activated protein C sensitivity ratio; APTT, activated partial
thromboplastin time; hCG, human chorionic gonadotrophin; PT, pro-
thrombin time; =, no effect; ↓, decreases; ↑, increases.

by OHSS showed a 100-fold increased risk of VTE, as opposed to the 5-fold increased
risk reported in the absence of OHSS.[2]

It is unclear, however, how OHSS increases this risk and why only a few women
seem to be predisposed to developing such complications. Whether thrombosis arises
as a result of blood modifications secondary to the clinical OHSS itself or as a consequence of the major changes in the steroid milieu induced by gonadotropin stimulation remains a matter of debate.

A specific role for biochemical hyperestrogenism associated with OHSS could be
postulated on the basis of the hyperestrogenic state that exists in pregnancy and in
users of oral contraceptives. However, as stated, the association between increased
estrogen levels and abnormal parameters of hemostasis during IVF is weak. Indeed,
no correlation was found between estrogen and changes in coagulation factors
observed in women with OHSS.[5] Moreover, thromboembolic events associated with
OHSS usually occur some time after the expected peak estradiol concentration.[9]

While the mechanism behind thrombogenesis during OHSS is uncertain, the increased risk that arises in association with this complication of IVF is clear. Careful monitoring and the judicious use of measures to avoid OHSS are particularly important in patients at risk of thrombosis.

In recent years a number of new strategies for reducing the incidence of OHSS have emerged. These include the use of GnRH antagonists rather than GnRH agonists to prevent premature luteinization, the use of GnRH agonists rather than hCG to trigger final oocyte maturation, the more liberal use of 'freeze all' cycles in which no fresh embryo transfer is carried out in the stimulated cycle, and the use of dopamine agonists to reduce symptoms. These strategies have been reviewed in the context of reducing VTE risk by Nelson.[10] Adequate hydration and thromboprophylaxis during treatment for OHSS are vital if life-threatening complications are to be avoided.

Preparing the Patient for IVF Treatment: Assess the Risk

All patients proceeding to IVF treatment should be individually assessed for their risk of thrombotic complications. Women who should be considered at increased risk include those with congenital or acquired thrombophilias, those who develop OHSS, those over 40 years of age and smokers (Table 2.2).

Congenital thrombophilias are a group of inherited disorders that include deficiencies in protein C, protein S and antithrombin; resistance to APC due to a point mutation (Arg506Gln) in the factor V gene (the factor V Leiden mutation); and a 677T polymorphism in the methylenetetrahydrofolate reductase gene (*MTHFR* 677T). Resistance to APC is an autosomal dominant trait caused by a mutation in the coagulation factor V gene. This mutation results in a replacement of arginine residue 506 with a glutamine at one of the factor V cleavage sites for APC. The factor V Leiden mutation that results in APC resistance has a high prevalence of 4–5% in Caucasians but is rare among Asians and Africans.

The prevalence of hyperhomocysteinemia in individuals with venous thrombosis has also been found to be high, and this represents an additional independent risk factor for DVT. A cause of moderate hyperhomocysteinemia is a relatively frequent mutation in the gene encoding 5,10-methylenetetrahydrofolate reductase (*MTHFR*).

In a study of women hospitalized for severe OHSS, 85% had one or more positive markers of thrombophilia compared with 27% of control subjects who had undergone IVF without developing severe OHSS.[11] The prevalence of *MTHFR* 677T and antithrombin and protein S deficiencies, but not the antiphospholipid syndrome or protein C deficiency, was significantly increased in women with severe OHSS.

TABLE 2.2

When to Consider Thromboprophylaxis

- Previous deep venous thrombosis (DVT)
- Ovarian hyperstimulation syndrome (OHSS) requiring hospital admission
- When antithrombin deficiency is present
- When other acquired or hereditary thrombophilias are present in combination with other risk factors such as age over 40 years and/or smoking
- When multiple risk factors such as high BMI, poor mobility, and smoking are identified.

Consistent with previous reports, all the clinically significant thrombotic events reported in this study occurred in women with more than one marker of thrombophilia.

Several case reports have been published describing women who developed venous thrombosis during IVF treatment and who were found to be APC resistant. However, of 31 women with factor V Leiden or factor II A20210 mutation undergoing IVF, none developed a thrombotic event during ovulation induction. In contrast, the combination of age > 39 years and plasma total homocysteine (tHcy) > 97.5th centile conferred a risk of thrombotic events 14–15-fold higher. The authors also assessed the prevalence of acquired thrombophilias in this cohort and found 5% tested positive for lupus anticoagulant.[12]

Acquired thrombophilias include the antiphospholipid syndrome, which is the presence of anticardiolipin antibodies or circulating lupus anticoagulants, deficiencies of antithrombin and protein S and acquired protein C resistance.

Prior VTE, Age and Obesity

Women with a previous episode of VTE are at greatly increased risk for recurrence, particularly when exposed to high-risk conditions. In a case-control study, patients with a history of VTE were around 16 times more likely to develop a new episode during a subsequent high-risk period compared with patients without a history of VTE or pulmonary embolism (PE).[13]

Patients aged > 40 years are at significantly increased risk of VTE, and obesity has long been cited as a risk factor for VTE. While risk may be increased, the association appears to be weak. The implications of obesity in IVF treatment are dealt with in detail in Chapter 8.

Screening for Thrombophilias

There is currently little evidence to support universal screening for thrombophilia in pregnancy or prior to IVF for the prevention of VTE.

However, screening for thrombophilia should be considered in women with a history of recurrent miscarriage or personal or family history of VTE. Thrombophilia is associated with a high risk of developing OHSS, and this has been proposed as an additional reason for screening for thrombophilia in women with a family or personal history of thrombosis prior to undergoing ovarian stimulation and in women who have developed OHSS. However, one study failed to show an increase in the prevalence of thrombophilia in women with severe OHSS, and the cost-effectiveness of screening for thrombophilias in this context of IVF could not be demonstrated.[14]

Screening for thrombophilias should include plasma antithrombin, proteins S and C, antiphospholipid antibodies, and testing for factor V Leiden mutation and *MTHFR* 677T.

Management of the IVF Cycle

Avoid OHSS

Patients deemed to be at additional risk of thrombosis should be advised as to the importance of avoiding the development of OHSS. Milder stimulation protocols in combination with a reduced dose of hCG (5000 IU or less) for triggering final oocyte maturation may reduce the risk without compromising chances of pregnancy. Judicious use of 'coasting' and the use of progesterone rather than hCG for luteal support have been shown to reduce the risk of OHSS.

However, the use of GnRH antagonists to prevent premature luteinization rather than GnRH agonists has been shown to significantly reduce the risk of OHSS and should be the first choice co-treatment in women at risk of DVT. Moreover, using GnRH antagonists rather than agonists makes it possible to avoid exposing the patient to a bolus of hCG to trigger final oocyte maturation by replacing this with a single dose of GnRH agonist. This has been shown to result in adequate oocyte maturation, but additional luteal support is required. This approach significantly reduces the risk of OHSS and should be considered in high-responding patients with risk factors of VTE. The risk of OHSS can be effectively removed if all embryos resulting from the stimulation cycle are frozen for later transfer, as it is implantation of an embryo in a woman at risk of OHSS which drives the ongoing hormonal stimulation which can lead to life-threatening complications.

Thromboprophylaxis

The decision whether or not to prescribe thromboprophylaxis in a given patient will depend on an individual assessment of the risk/benefit of treatment in each patient. The presence or absence of the risk factors addressed in this chapter should direct treatment. Table 2.2 summarises clinical situations in which thromboprophylaxis should be considered.

Although thromboprophylaxis is often commenced with ovarian stimulation, it is probably not necessary at that stage. Given the rarity of VTE prior to hCG, and the increased risk of significant intra-abdominal bleeding that may occur following oocyte pickup, medical thromboprophylaxis can be delayed until after this procedure has been carried out. However, most practitioners will wish to start prophylaxis with ovarian stimulation, stop for 24 hours prior to oocyte pickup and then reinstitute treatment. In a study of 74 patients thus treated, no case of perioperative bleeding was reported.[15] Low-molecular-weight heparin (LMWH) remains the first-line pharmacological method and recent studies indicate that a dose of at least 5000 U of dalteparin or equivalent is probably optimal. However, at a low body weight (<50 kg or body mass index [BMI] < 20 kg/m^2), lower doses may be required (e.g. 20 mg enoxaparin or 2500 IU dalteparin daily), and in obese patients (BMI > 30), higher doses may be required.

The platelet count should be checked before and 1 week after commencing LMWH to detect heparin-induced thrombocytopenia. The optimal duration of thromboprophylaxis remains unclear. However there is a consensus emerging from the published literature that thromboprophylaxis should be continued until either 6 weeks after embryo transfer or 6 weeks after discharge from hospital if OHSS arises. In those who conceive, longer-term prophylaxis may be indicated.

Low-dose (60–75 mg) aspirin has been widely used in pregnancy to prevent pre-eclampsia and in IVF in attempt to improve implantation. It is well tolerated and has few side effects. The effectiveness of aspirin as a thromboprophylactic agent in pregnancy and IVF remains to be established, but it is likely to be less than that of LMWH. In women with hyperhomocysteinemia, the risk of developing VTE may be reduced by folic acid supplementation.

Women who have suffered previous episodes of VTE known to have an underlying cause may present for IVF already under long-term anticoagulant therapy with warfarin. Normally women who conceive should be switched to LMWH before 6 weeks gestation to avoid the risks of coumarin embryopathy. In women undergoing IVF this switch can be instituted prior to commencing ovarian stimulation. This allows the risk of bleeding at oocyte pickup to be reduced by stopping LMWH 24 hours prior to the procedure, restarting treatment on the evening after oocyte retrieval. Advised dosages of LMWH in this case are enoxaparin 0.5–1 mg/kg 12 hourly or dalteparin 5 100 IU/kg 12 hourly, with an aim of achieving anti-Xa levels of 0.7–1.0.[16]

Should a patient develop a higher VTE, therapeutic doses of LMWH are required. Enoxaparin 1 mg/kg 12 hourly or dalteparin 90 IU/kg 12 hourly are advised. Specialist advice will be required to determine the duration of therapy, but normally a minimum of 6 months of therapeutic doses is advised, followed by prophylactic doses continuing until 6 weeks post-partum.[16]

Post-IVF Follow-Up

Clinical reports of VTE occurring following IVF treatment usually report the event occurring in early pregnancy, between 5 and 10 weeks after hCG administration. Many reported cases of VTE following IVF described it occurring in sites other than the lower limb, but this may simply reflect publication bias. The jugular vein appears to be a relatively frequent site. The majority of thromboses occurring here were associated with hormonal ovarian stimulation.[17]

Recent case reports have demonstrated the value of ultrasound in the diagnosis of both lower-extremity, upper-extremity and neck vein DVT.

For more information on both the further management of VTE and of bleeding disorders in the context of IVF, readers are referred to the work of Nelson and Greer.[16]

Summary of Management Options

1. DVT occurring after IVF is a rare but potentially life-threatening complication of IVF.

2. All patients beginning IVF should be subjected to an individual risk assessment prior to commencing treatment.

3. There is little evidence that increased estradiol levels underlie the increased risk associated with IVF treatment.

4. In the period following hCG administration, considerable changes in the coagulation and fibrinolytic systems are observed.

5. Screening for thrombophilias should be considered in women who have had a previous thrombotic event or a family history of thrombosis, in women who have developed OHSS and in women over 40 years of age.

6. Thromboprophylaxis should be considered in women with a previous DVT, in women who develop OHSS and in women over 40 years with a thrombophilia. In addition, women who develop serious infections or immobilization due to surgery should receive thromboprophylaxis.

7. Compression stockings and LMWH constitute first-line thromboprophylaxis, and this should continue for 6 weeks in non-pregnant women.

REFERENCES

1. Hansen AT, Kesmodel US, Juul S, Hvas AM. No evidence that assisted reproduction increases the risk of thrombosis: A Danish national cohort study. *Hum Reprod* 2012 May; 27(5): 1499–503.
2. Rova K, Passmark H, Lindqvist PG. Venous thromboembolism in relation to in vitro fertilization: An approach to determining the incidence and increase in risk in successful cycles. *Fertil Steril* 2012; 97: 95–100.
3. Tilney ML, Griffiths HJ, Edwards EA. Natural history of major venous thrombosis of the upper extremity. *Arch Surg* 1970; 101: 792–6.
4. Lox C, Canez M, DeLeon F, et al. Hyperestrogenism induced by menotropins alone or in conjunction with leuprolide acetate in in-vitro fertilization cycles: The impact on hemostasis. *Fertil Steril* 1995; 63: 566–70.
5. Biron C, Galtier-Dereure F, Rabesandratana H, et al. Hemostasis parameters during ovarian stimulation for in-vitro fertilization: results of a prospective study. *Fertil Steril* 1997; 67: 104–9.
6. Lox C, Canez M, Prien S. The influence of hyperestrogenism during *in vitro* fertilization on the fibrunolytic mechanism. *Int J Fertil* 1998; 43: 34–9.
7. Curvers J, Nap AW, Thomassen MC, et al. Effect of in-vitro fertilization treatment and subsequent pregnancy on the protein C pathway. *Br J Haematol* 2001; 115: 400–7.
8. Kodama H, Fukuda J, Karube H, Matsui T, et al. Status of the coagulation and fibrino-lytic systems in ovarian hyperstimulation syndrome. *Fertil Steril* 1996; 66: 417–24.
9. Stewart JA, Hamilton PJ, Murdoch AP. Thromboembolic disease associated with ovarian stimulation and assisted conception techniques. *Hum Reprod* 1997; 12: 2167–73.
10. Nelson SM. Venous thrombosis during assisted reproduction: novel risk reduction strategies. *Thromb Res* 2013 Jan; 131 Suppl 1: S1–3.
11. Dulitzky M, Cohen SB, Inbal A, et al. Increased prevalance of thrombophilia among women with severe ovarian hyperstimulation syndrome. *Fertil Steril* 2002; 77: 463–7.
12. Grandone E, Colaizzo D, Cappuci F, et al. Age and homocysteine plasma levels are risk factors for thrombotic complications after ovarian stimulation. *Hum Reprod* 2004; 19: 1796–9.
13. Samama MM. An epidemiologic study of risk factors for deep vein thrombosis in medical outpatients: The Sirius study. *Arch Intern Med* 2000; 160: 3415–20.
14. Fábregues F, Tàssies D, Reverter JC, et al. Prevalence of thrombophilia in women with severe ovarian hyperstimulation syndrome and cost-effectiveness of screening. *Fertil Steril* 2004; 81: 989–95.
15. Yinon Y, Pauzner R, Dulitzky M, Elizur SE, Dor J, Shulman A. Safety of IVF under anticoagulant therapy in patients at risk for thrombo-embolic events. *Reprod Biomed Online* 2006 Mar; 12(3): 354–8.
16. Nelson S, Greer I. The patient at risk from thrombosis and bleeding disorders. In: Macklon, Steegers and Greer, editors. *Textbook of Periconceptional Medicine,* Informa, London 2009.
17. Fleming T, Sacks G, Nasser J. Internal jugular vein thrombosis following ovarian hyperstimulation syndrome. *Aust N Z J Obstet Gynaecol* 2012 Feb; 52(1): 87–90.

3

The Patient with Hyperprolactinaemia

AN Andersen, MP Lauritsen, and M Krog

CONTENTS

KEY WORDS: *hyperprolactinaemia, IVF, pregnancy*

Background

The availability of effective treatment of hyperprolactinaemic anovulatory infertility pre-dated the emergence of in vitro fertilization (IVF). The use of dopamine agonists such as bromocriptine entered clinical practice in the early 1970s.

Hyperprolactinaemic patients typically present with anovulatory infertility due to either a disturbed hypothalamic pulsatile gonatrophin-releasing hormone (GnRH) release or anatomical processes/defects in the pituitary, directly inhibiting follicle-stimulating hormone (FSH) and luteinizing hormone (LH) release from the gonadotrophic cells. The ovarian reserve is normal, and hyperprolactinaemic patients with anovulation respond well to treatment with dopamine agonists such as bromocriptine or cabergoline, and the great majority menstruate, ovulate and conceive when the prolactin level is normalized.[1] A few hypogonadotrophic patients with macroprolactinomas and some with insensitivity to dopamine agonists will not ovulate and conceive after dopamine agonist treatment, but these patients respond well to ovulation induction with exogenous gonatrophins. Thus, only a small fraction of infertile hyperprolactinaemic anovulatory patients needs treatment with IVF, either due to contributing causes of infertility, such as male or tubal factors, or due to lack of conception after several attempts at ovulation induction.

There is no specific literature on the management of anovulatory hyperprolactinaemic patients in IVF, but this chapter summarises key aspects that reproductive endocrinologists should consider before and after exposing patients to treatment.

Defining Hyperprolactinaemia in Patients with Infertility

Before classifying any infertile patient as having clinically important hyperprolactinaemia, a number of issues should be clarified (Table 3.1):

1. Prolactin is a stress hormone, and the release of prolactin is as sensitive to stress factors as cortisol. Thus, marginally elevated prolactin levels are frequently found in normally ovulatory women and when screening infertile patients. The mere stress of a pelvic examination may induce an elevated prolactin level in many patients for a couple of hours, and an endometrial biopsy may cause a 3- to 5-fold prolactin elevation for several hours in the majority of women.

   Any elevated prolactin measurement should therefore be repeated, and care should be taken to obtain the serum sample under basal conditions.[1] Fluctuating prolactin levels, including values within the normal ranges, are typically stress related, and with no reproductive consequences.

2. Some women with normal ovulatory cycles present with apparent hyperprolactinaemia due to the release of macroprolactin, a polymer of the molecule that is less bioactive than the monomer.[2] The presence of macroprolactinaemia can be assessed using special assays, and it is recommended that these be performed in cases of asymptomatic hyperprolactinaemia.[1] Such asymptomatic hyperprolactinaemic patients typically found during screening would not need special attention as long as they remain ovulatory.

TABLE 3.1

Considerations before IVF Treatment in a Hyperprolactinaemic Patient

Before Entering IVF Treatment	
Is the diagnosis of persistent hyperprolactinaemic anovulation established?	Exclude clinically insignificant hyperprolactinaemia induced by stressful sampling conditions, medications and minor prolactin elevations in patients with anovulation due to PCOS.
Does the patient have a pituitary macroprolactinoma/macroadenoma (>10 mm)?	The higher the prolactin level, the higher the risk of a macroprolactinoma, but serum prolactin cannot be used to exclude a larger pituitary adenoma/prolactinoma. Pituitary imaging is needed.
Does the patient also have impairments in the thyroid and/or adrenal hormone secretions?	The ART specialist should consult the endocrinologist. Thyroid and/or adrenal substitution therapy should be implemented before IVF.
Has the patient been given an adequate number of ovulation induction cycles with dopamine agonist/gonadotrophins?	Unless well-defined additional causes of infertility are present, 6–9 ovulatory cycles should have been done before entering an IVF program. If dopamine agonist insensitive, these patients are fully responsive to exogenous gonadotrophins.

3. Anovulatory infertile patients often have polycystic ovary syndrome (PCOS), and some of these patients may present with marginally elevated prolactin.[3] It should therefore be determined whether the primary disorder of any hyperprolactinaemic anovulatory patient is PCOS, or whether the anovulation is primarily due to hyperprolactinaemia. For this purpose standard diagnostic criteria for the two conditions should be applied, and anti-Müllerian hormone (AMH) may additionally be used to discriminate between the two conditions.[4] AMH level reflects the difference in ovarian reserve between PCOS patients and patients with isolated elevated prolactin (increased vs. normal).

4. A number of drugs cause hyperprolactinaemia. Drug-induced hyperprolactinaemia should thus be excluded.[1]

Diagnostic Assessment before IVF

The hyperprolactinaemic patients most often have (1) idiopathic hyperprolactinaemia, (2) a microprolactinoma or (3) a macroprolactinoma (>10 mm). However, a large number of rare disorders may also cause hyperprolactinaemia. These conditions are related to hypothalamic-pituitary stalk damage (granulomas, Rathke's cysts, craniopharyngiomas, germinomas, meningiomas, hypothalamic metastases), the pituitary itself (acromegaly, lymphocytic hypophysitis, non-prolactin-secreting macroadenomas) or various disorders (hypothyroidism, neurogenic crest-related disorders, chronic renal failure or cirrhosis). For a review, see the work of Melmed et al.[1]

Based on this complex pathophysiology, there are several reasons hyperprolactinaemic patients should be investigated by an endocrinologist before IVF is performed.

Firstly, even though several of the diagnoses mentioned are rare, some may have serious health consequences and should be diagnosed and appropriately treated, either medically or surgically. The majority of patients with prolactinomas (prolactin-secreting adenomas of the anterior pituitary) have microprolactinomas, and they rarely progress to macroprolactinomas. However, a proportion do harbour macroprolactinomas (>10 mm), and here, the key consideration is the size of the prolactinoma and whether there is suprasellar growth with the known risk of impaired visual field due to compression of the optic nerves.

Secondly, processes like macroprolactinomas, pituitary macroadenomas or sequelae after pituitary surgery may impair pituitary function and cause deficiencies not only in the hypothalamic-pituitary-ovarian axis but also in the secretion of TSH (thyroid-stimulating hormone) and adrenocorticotrophic hormone (ACTH). As a normal thyroid and adrenal function is crucial for a normal pregnancy, lack of substitution of the TRH (thyrotropin-releasing hormone), TSH and thyroid hormone axis, especially during the first and second trimester, may have consequences for fetal health and development. Patients with macroprolactinomas should thus be fully investigated, and if substitution therapy is needed, this should be initiated before IVF.

Impact of the Disease on Pregnancy

Except for the rare cases where hyperprolactinaemia is related to systemic diseases, hyperprolactinaemia is a central disorder that does not influence ovarian reserve or the response to exogenous gonadotropins. Luteal function is not influenced by hyperprolactinaemia, as it has been shown that dopamine agonist treatment can be withdrawn as soon as ovulation occurs with no influence on the luteal phase. When the pregnancy is established, hyperprolactinaemia will not influence the course of pregnancy, but as discussed in the following material, the pregnancy may have consequences for the hyperprolactinaemia.

Is IVF Needed?

Before a decision is made to do IVF in a hyperprolactinaemic patient, we recommend that the ART (assisted reproductive technology) specialist should make a final critical evaluation of whether IVF is really needed. The fact that 80–90% of patients with hyperprolactinaemia conceive *in vivo* following dopamine agonist therapy should be considered.[1,5] However, some patients seem rather resistant to dopamine agonists, as their prolactin is not normalized even after high doses of cabergoline treatment.[5] When ovulatory cycles and conception are not achieved, the possibility of traditional gonatrophin therapy for ovulation induction remains unless a well-defined tubal or severe male factor is present (Table 3.1).

Preparing the Patient for IVF

The choice of protocols and drugs for controlled ovarian stimulation in IVF is not clarified in literature, but as summarised in Table 3.2, our recommendations would be the following:

1. The patients should be continuously treated with either bromocriptine or cabergoline, the two drugs for which most data are available on safety in pregnancy. Other dopamine agonists should not be used for these patients.

TABLE 3.2

Considerations Regarding Controlled Ovarian Stimulation for IVF in a Hyperprolactinaemic Patient

Controlled Ovarian Stimulation for IVF	
Are hyperprolactinaemic patients expected to have a normal ovarian response to gonadotrophins?	Yes. Hyperprolactinaemia induces anovulation through central mechanisms, not interfering directly with the ovaries.
Does the patient need dopamine agonist before and during controlled ovarian stimulation for IVF?	It is recommended to use either bromocriptine or cabergoline. The patients who menstruate and ovulate on this therapy can enter either a long agonist or an antagonist protocol.
If ovulatory cycles are not induced by dopamine agonist therapy, how should the controlled ovarian stimulation be started?	If oestrogens are low and the endometrial lining is thin, controlled ovarian stimulation can be started without a withdrawal bleeding.
Is there any FSH preparation that should be preferred?	There are no data on this but a preparation with LH or LH activity may be preferred in patients with relative hypogonadotropism.

2. In patients who menstruate and ovulate on bromocriptine or cabergoline, a long agonist or short antagonist protocol could be used according to the routine of the clinic.

3. If the patient remains anovulatory on dopamine agonist treatment, there are two ways of initiating the controlled ovarian stimulation. One possibility is to use a simple oestrogen-progestogen substitution followed by gonatrophin therapy in the GnRH antagonist protocol from day 3 of bleeding. Alternatively, in cases where serum oestradiol is low and sonography of the endometrium shows a thin lining, the antagonist protocol could start on an arbitrary day. As these patients are already "downregulated", it is not necessary to use the long GnRH agonist protocol.

4. In terms of choice of FSH, we would add LH or use a preparation containing "LH activity" in order to achieve adequate oestrogenisation. As the ovarian reserve is normal in hyperprolactinaemic patients,[4] these patients should also receive the standard doses of FSH applied in the clinic.

Management in Early Pregnancy

If a hyperprolactinaemic patient achieves a pregnancy, there are a number of considerations (Table 3.3).

When to Withdraw Dopamine Agonist Therapy

The Endocrine Society clinical practise guidelines recommend that bromocriptine or cabergoline should be withdrawn as soon as the pregnancy is confirmed,[1]

TABLE 3.3

Considerations When a Hyperprolactinaemic Patient Becomes Pregnant after IVF

The Patient Is Pregnant after ART	
Should bromocriptine or carbergoline be withdrawn when the pregnancy is diagnosed?	Yes. Even though it seems safe to give these drugs, the recommendation is to withdraw, and no negative effects of this are apparent.
What is the risk of clinically significant enlargement of a pituitary prolactinoma/adenoma during pregnancy?	<2% in microprolactinomas. 20–25% in macroprolactinomas.
What is the key parameter to follow during pregnancy?	Clinical symptoms, headache, visual field disturbances and examination of visual field defects. Routine imaging like MRI is not indicated. Routine serial controls of prolactin levels are not recommended.
What is the prognosis in case of symptoms due to growth of a prolactinoma?	The prognosis is good as re-initiation of dopamine agonist therapy normally shrinks prolactinomas rapidly.
What is the prognosis after a pregnancy?	Good, and some patients even experience lower serum prolactin, and there is a good prognosis for spontaneous recovery/remission after a pregnancy.
Can hyperprolactinaemic patients breastfeed?	Yes; no concerns.

which is usually in gestation week 4 in pregnancies after IVF. Bromocriptine crosses the placenta in humans, and cabergoline is known to cross the placenta in animals, so the recommendations are based on the general precautions for all drugs used during organogenesis and fetal growth. However, some patients, typically those who have macroprolactinomas, have taken the drug throughout pregnancy, apparently without any adverse effects on the fetus or mother.[1,6]

When the dopamine agonist is withdrawn, the prolactin level will immediately rise, but as the effects of hyperprolactinaemia are mediated in the hypothalamus, this rise in serum prolactin does not seem to interfere with corpora lutea of early pregnancies, and the miscarriage rates do not seem to be increased.[7]

Is Bromocriptine or Cabergoline Teratogenic?

The available data on the use of bromocriptine or cabergoline in pregnancy are reassuring in terms of safety. The literature reports data from more than 5000 infants who were exposed to bromocriptine during early pregnancy, and the incidences of miscarriages or congenital malformations are not increased.[7] In terms of cabergoline the literature is less extensive, but available data from several studies[5,8] indicate that this drug can also be safely used in patients who wish to conceive. As reviewed by Molitch,[7] data from 350 cases indicated that there is no increased risk of miscarriage, preterm birth or congenital abnormalities.

Impact of Pregnancy on the Hyperprolactinaemia

The prolactin-secreting lactotrophic cells of the anterior pituitary are sensitive to oestrogens during pregnancy, leading to a physiological enlargement of the anterior pituitary and a 10-fold rise in serum prolactin. These effects are believed to be due to the rise in circulating oestrogens causing hyperplasia of the lactotrophic cells during gestation. The endocrine changes in pregnancy may also influence the pituitary in hyperprolactinaemic patients, and two issues should thus be considered if a hyperprolactinaemic patient becomes pregnant:

1. What is the risk that a prolactinoma will expand to such an extent that it may be of clinical significance?
2. Will the pregnancy change the prognosis for the mother?

The risk of clinically significant tumor enlargement is highly dependent on whether the prolactinoma is a micro- or macroprolactinoma. Based on a review of 376 pregnant women with microprolactinomas from 19 studies, the risk estimate is that only 6/376 (1.3%) of the microprolactinomas caused significant clinical problems (headache or visual disturbances or both). In contrast, based on the same series, 20/86 (23.2%) of patients with macroprolactinomas who had not been exposed to pituitary surgery had symptomatic pituitary enlargement. Thus, almost 1 of 4 of the macroprolactinoma patients needed intervention in the form of either surgery or re-initiation of dopamine agonist therapy during pregnancy (for review see Molitch[7]).

The data show that the pretreatment tumor size (micro- versus macroprolactinomas) is critical in terms of risk of clinical complications induced by the pregnancy.

The message to the clinician is therefore that all patients with prolactinomas should be guided to consult their doctor in terms of headache and/or visual disturbances.

During pregnancy the changes in prolactin levels in hyperprolactinaemic patients follow an unpredictable pattern. In some patients a marked rise in serum prolactin is found which may be associated with prolactinoma growth, whereas in other patients serum levels decline as the pregnancy progresses.[6] However, there is no consistent pattern that may allow the clinician to predict whether or not a prolactinoma is expanding. In the latest guideline by the Endocrine Society of the United States,[1] it is not recommended to follow serum prolactin changes during gestation. Thus, from the second trimester and onwards, the clinician must rely on clinical symptoms and visual field examinations of the pregnant patients. In the same guideline, it is recommended not to use magnetic resonance imaging (MRI) routinely, but only to apply imaging techniques in cases with clinical suspicion of tumor expansion.

If a prolactinoma causes symptomatic enlargement during the course of pregnancy, the treatment would typically be to re-initiate dopamine agonist therapy, which will usually cause rapid shrinkage of the prolactinoma and clearance of the clinical symptoms.

Hyperprolactinaemic mothers can lactate as others, with no restrictions in terms of breastfeeding.

The final question is whether a pregnancy may change the long-term prognosis for the mother. Indeed, regression of the hyperprolactinaemic state is rather common after a pregnancy, and complete remission occurs in some cases. There is no available evidence that the long-term prognosis will be worse after a pregnancy induced by IVF treatment.

REFERENCES

1. Melmed S, Casanueva FF, Hoffman AR, et al. Diagnosis and treatment of hyperprolactinemia: An Endocrine Society clinical practise guideline. *J Clin Endocrinol Metab* 2001; 96: 273–88.
2. Andersen AN, Pedersen H, Djursing H, et al. Bioactivity of prolactin in a woman with an excess of large molecular size prolactin, persistent hyperprolactinemia and spontaneous conception. *Fertil Steril* 1982; 38: 625–8.
3. Su HW, Chen CM, Chou SY, et al. Polycystic ovary syndrome or hyperprolactinaemia: a study of mild hyperprolactinaemia. *Gynecol Endocrinol* 2011; 27: 55–62.
4. Li HW, Anderson RA, Yeung WS, et al. Evaluation of serum antimullerian hormone and inhibin B concentrations in the differential diagnosis of secondary oligoamenorrhea. *Fertil Steril* 2011; 96: 774–9.
5. Ono M, Miki N, Amano M, et al. Individualized high-dose cabergoline therapy for hyperprolactinemic infertility in women with micro- and macroprolactinomas. *J Clin Endocrinol Metab* 2010; 95: 2672–9.
6. Andersen AN, Starup J, Tabor A, et al. The possible prognostic value of prolactin increment during pregnancy in hyperprolactinaemic patients. *Acta Endocrinologica* 1983; 102: 1–5.
7. Molitch ME. Pituitary disorders during pregnancy. *Endocrinol Metab Clin North Am* 2006; 35(1): 99–116.
8. Colao A, Abs R, Bárcena DG, et al. Pregnancy outcomes following cabergoline treatment: extended results from a 12-year observational study. *Clin Endocrinol* 2008; 68: 66–71.

4

The Patient with Autoimmune Disease

D Galliano, A Pellicer, and J Bellver

CONTENTS

KEY WORDS: *systemic lupus erythematosus, antiphospholipid syndrome, ovarian stimulation, infertility, IVF, pregnancy*

Background

Systemic Lupus Erythematosus

Systemic lupus erythematosus (SLE) is an inflammatory autoimmune disease characterized by the production of autoantibodies and the presence of clinical manifestations affecting multiple organs.[1] SLE is a chronic disorder with an unpredictable course, alternating between periods of flares with remissions. The prevalence ranges from 20 to 150 cases per 100,000 persons and appears to be increasing due to better diagnosis and survival. The disease occurs nine times more often in women than in men, especially in women of childbearing age, and tends to be more severe among the black population. Due to earlier diagnosis and advances in treatments, the current life expectancy of such patients has improved to approximately 80% at 15 years. Even with these advances, however, one-third of SLE-related deaths in the United States occur in patients younger than 45 years due to active disease, cardiovascular complications, or infections secondary to immunosuppressive treatment.

SLE etiology is not fully known, but a strong genetic component has been shown to play a key role in the predisposition of this disease. Many genes that may contribute to lupus have been identified in families where multiple members have the disease, with eight susceptibility loci located in chromosomes 1, 2, 4, 6, 12, and 16.

TABLE 4.1

Classification Clinical and Laboratory Criteria for SLE

1. Malar rash
2. Discoid rash
3. Photosensitivity
4. Oral ulcers
5. Arthritis
6. Pleuritis or pericarditis
7. Renal disorder
8. Neurologic disorder
9. Hematologic disorder
10. Immunologic disorder
11. Antinuclear antibodies

Source: Adapted from Bellver J, Pellicer A. *Fertil Steril* 2009 Dec;92(6):1803–10.

Note: Four of the 11 criteria are needed for the formal diagnosis.

Genes of the major histocompatibility complex (MHC), particularly HLA-A1, B8, and DR3, have been linked to SLE, as well as certain single-nucleotide polymorphisms (SNPs) that are associated with its clinical manifestations.[2]

Ninety percent of patients affected with SLE are women, and in genetically manipulated mice the presence of two X chromosomes increases the severity of the disorder, demonstrating the strong link between SLE and gender.[2] Environmental factors, such as smoking and exposure to ultraviolet radiation, have also been associated with SLE, as well as drugs such as procainamide, hydralazine and quinidine. Epstein–Barr virus (EBV) infection may also trigger lupus, as suggested by higher viral load in patients with SLE than in controls, as well as the inability of CD8+ T cells to control EBV-infected B cells. Genetic, epigenetic, environmental, and hormonal factors contribute to the expression of inflammation and damage to vital organs and tissues, especially joints, kidneys, skin, liver, and vessel walls, with varying degrees of severity, ranging from dermatologic and musculoskeletal symptoms to anemia, serositis, nephritis, and neuropsychiatric disorders.

Due to the clinical heterogeneity of the disease, 11 clinical or laboratory criteria have been established by the American College of Rheumatology, with a minimum of 4 criteria required for the correct diagnosis of SLE (95% specificity and 85% sensitivity) (Table 4.1).

Treatment of the disease includes nonsteroidal anti-inflammatory medications, antimalarial agents, glucocorticoids and immunosuppressive/cytotoxic drugs, such as hydroxychloroquine, azathioprine, methotrexate and cyclophosphamide.

Antiphospholipid Syndrome

Antiphospholipid syndrome (APS) is a prothrombotic disorder characterized by pregnancy morbidity and the presence of persistent antiphospholipid antibodies (aPLs).[3] APS predominantly affects women, with a mean age at diagnosis of 31 years (15–85 years). Although any tissue can be affected, the veins of the lower limbs and the cerebral arterials are the most common sites of venous and arterial thrombosis, respectively, with the risk of thrombosis ranging from 0.5–30%. Catastrophic APS is rare and presents high mortality due to multiorgan failure. Although several pathogenic mechanisms explaining how aPLs cause thrombosis have been proposed, the relationship between aPLs and the wide variety of clinical findings – ranging from normal pregnancies to thromboembolism or obstetric complications – remains unclear.[4]

The revised classification criteria for APS (2006) include specific autoantibodies as a needed component of the diagnosis. The persistence of more than 12 weeks of high titers of anti–β2-glycoprotein I (ab2GP1), or immunoglobulin (Ig) M and/or IgG anticardiolipin antibodies (ACAs) or lupus anticoagulant (LAC), is required. A diagnosis of APS is made if at least one of these clinical criteria and one of the laboratory criteria are met. The clinical criteria include vascular thrombosis and pregnancy morbidity, defined as recurrent early miscarriage, fetal death, preterm delivery (< 34 weeks) caused by placental insufficiency or preeclampsia, and small size for gestational age (birth weight < 5th percentile). Even if aPLs are closely related to pregnancy complications, no consensus exists regarding which specific autoantibodies are more predictive of adverse obstetric outcome. Indeed, some retrospective studies have suggested that the simultaneous presence of LAC, ACAs, and ab2GP1 is the best predictor of at-risk patients; SLE or recurrent pregnancy loss (RPL) have been suggested by other investigators to have predictive power; and a recent prospective, multicenter study has shown that LAC is the only component of triple positivity that is strictly predictive.[5]

Impact of SLE and APS on IVF and Pregnancy

Fertility seems to be normal in women with SLE, except in cases of severe disease and ovarian failure secondary to cyclophosphamide (CTX) therapy, which is reported in up to 70% of patients. In this regard, ovarian or oocyte cryopreservation before receiving alkylating agents employed in SLE should be recommended to preserve future fertility.

Even though some retrospective studies have in the past suggested a relationship between antiphospholipid antibodies, infertility and poor assisted reproductive technique (ART) outcome, more recent studies, including from our own group, have not detected a higher prevalence of lupus anticoagulant or ACAs in infertile women compared to fertile egg donors. Indeed, neither the routine screening in the infertile population nor the anticoagulant therapy in the presence of antiphospholipid antibodies appears justified since such antibodies do not seem to affect ART outcome.

Pregnancy represents a dangerous period in which the rates of obstetrical complications are high, particularly the unexplained death of normal fetuses and recurrent spontaneous abortions prior to the 10th week of gestation, and the premature birth of neonates prior to the 34th week of gestation due to eclampsia, most often when antiphospholipid antibodies or renal disease are present. Fetal congenital heart block is observed in 2–4.5% of SLE pregnancies, primarily when positive anti-Ro and/or anti-La antibodies are present and may lead to fetal death. Moreover, pulmonary hypertension shown by over 14% of patients with lupus is associated with a high risk of maternal death.

Given these data, for women affected by SLE and APS, IVF seems to be safe when the disease is in clinical remission and prophylactic anticoagulant therapy is administered. Pregnancy should be discouraged in patients with disease inactivity

TABLE 4.2

Clinical Situations in which Ovarian Stimulation Should Be Discouraged in Women with SLE

Acute flare (and the following 6–12 months)
Pulmonary hypertension or arterial hypertension
Valvulopathy or heart disease
Previous thromboembolism
Severe renal disease
Antiphospholipid syndrome and anti-Ro/anti-La antibodies

Source: Adapted from Bellver J, Pellicer A. *Fertil Steril* 2009 Dec;92(6):1803–10.

less than 6–12 months, arterial and pulmonary hypertension, renal involvement, and antiphospholipid or anti-Ro/anti-La antibodies (Table 4.2).

Impact of IVF and Pregnancy on SLE and APS

Women with SLE and APS undergoing controlled ovarian hyperstimulation (COH) and IVF are at increased risk of hormone-associated flare and venous and arterial thromboembolism due to the hypercoagulable state induced by high serum estradiol (E2) concentrations, as well as enhanced risk of maternal and fetal complications. A planned and short COH with administration of prophylactic therapy, during a remission phase of the disease, especially with corticosteroids and anticoagulants, increases the safety of the procedure and reduces the risk of these complications. Pregnancy may aggravate SLE in several ways, for instance, by increasing the likelihood of a flare, which occurs in late pregnancy or puerperium in 46.6% of cases; deteriorating renal function, especially in patients with hypertension, heavy proteinuria, or high serum creatinine concentration; and increasing the risk of maternal thrombosis, especially in the puerperium and when antiphospholipid antibodies are present.

Preparing the Patient for IVF

IVF physicians should be aware of the relationship between immunologic alterations and reproductive outcomes and therefore recommend thrombophilia screening, immunologic tests and genetic study to patients in the presence of RPL, chemical pregnancy losses, or two or three failed IVF cycles. According to the first recent world survey, the most ordered immunologic tests for RPL and repeated implantation failures (RIF) are ACAs, LAC, thyroid peroxidase antibody, and antinuclear antibody, as opposed to the less-frequently investigated NK assay, human leukocyte antigen study, Th1/Th2 study or immunophenotype assay.[6]

Moreover, as an increase in disease activity can occur during IVF, timing of pregnancy relative to SLE/APS activity has to be prudently considered, and accordingly a treatment process should be started only in selected patients.

Reproductive specialists should therefore be familiar with the impact of these disorders on IVF and pregnancy and carefully plan IVF by screening the patient for presence of autoantibodies and immune alterations, clinical inflammation, and hormonal dysfunction that may contribute to the complications mentioned. Indeed, after a prognosis of the disease established with prenatal counseling, COH and IVF should be realized only in well-selected patients free of these risk factors to make the treatment safe and successful. In such women, treatment with prophylactic/therapeutic actions does not increase complications during IVF, and the rates of live and healthy births are high, ranging from 66% to 85%.[7]

Management during IVF Treatment

It has been shown that oral contraceptives with high doses of oestrogen can induce or exacerbate the lupus activity, as well as the risk of venous and arterial thrombosis, particularly in the presence of APS. However, when the disease is inactive or stable, without high titres of antiphospholipid antibodies and negative LA, oral contraceptives with the lowest possible dose of ethinylestradiol may be administered. With respect to IVF, in SLE/APS women it is strongly advised to avoid ovarian hyperstimulation syndrome (OHSS) by employing strategies that include mild stimulation protocols, cycle cancellation, coasting, administration of GnRH agonists for oocyte retrieval, and embryo freezing, as well as single-embryo transfer[8] to reduce complications related to multiple pregnancies.

The natural cycle should be the first option in case of egg donation and transfer of frozen embryos. When estrogens are employed for endometrial preparation, less procoagulant natural estrogens should be considered to avoid the first-passage effect in the liver and should be administered transdermally rather than orally. Similarly, natural progesterone through vaginal administration is preferable to synthetic progesterone in order to avoid the first-passage effect (Table 4.3).

To reduce the risk of thrombosis and/or lupus flares, anticoagulation, corticosteroids, and immunosuppressants should be administered during and after ovarian stimulation.

TABLE 4.3

Guidelines for Ovarian Stimulation in Women with SLE and/or APS

1. Lowest dose of ethinylestradiol ($\leq$30 µg) in combined oral contraceptives if inactive or stable/moderate disease with no history of venous or arterial thrombosis, no history of lupus exacerbation with estrogens, no lupus anticoagulant, no high titres of any antiphospholipid antibody isotype (IgG > 40 GPL, IgM > 40 MPL, IgA > 50 APL)
2. Friendly ovarian stimulation
3. Avoid OHSS
4. SET
5. Coadjuvant therapy: anticoagulation, corticosteroids, immunosuppressants
6. Transfer of frozen embryos and ovum donation
   - natural cycles
   - natural estradiol
   - transdermal route
7. Luteal phase support
   - natural progesterone
   - vaginal route

Source: Adapted from Bellver J, Pellicer A. *Fertil Steril* 2009 Dec;92(6):1803–10.

Women with antiphospholipid antibodies and no history of thrombosis should be treated with heparin from the beginning of the luteal phase after embryo transfer, when the risk of thrombosis is increased, and not prior to ovum retrieval. In contrast, women with antiphospholipid antibodies who have a history of thrombosis should be switched from oral anticoagulant therapy to heparin from the beginning of the ovarian stimulation. In both cases, heparin should be stopped 12–24 hours prior to ovum retrieval to reduce bleeding complications, re-started 6–12 hours later, and then maintained until the day of the pregnancy test and continued in case of pregnancy. To avoid bleeding, low-dose aspirin should be considered and interrupted 5 to 7 days before oocyte retrieval. In women with only SLE and not APS, anticoagulation is not recommended, but cortico-steroids and immunosuppressants should be employed to reduce lupus flares, especially when gonadotropins are given.[8]

Management in Early Pregnancy

Pregnancy in patients with SLE/APS leads to an increased risk of maternal and fetal complications which require close monitoring with the involvement of experienced specialists. Despite the advances made in the management of these pregnancies, however, adverse outcomes, including preeclampsia, pregnancy loss, intrauterine growth restriction (IUGR), and prematurity, still remain frequent as well as placental ischemia due to poor vascularization and impairment of early placenta.

In order to prevent or promptly recognize these complications in early pregnancy, clinical and laboratory biomarkers have been investigated, but the current evidence has shown LAC to be the strongest factor predicting adverse pregnancy outcomes, especially thrombosis, in these women.[9,10] Therefore, because of this increased rate of complications, early pregnancy must be strictly followed up, with strong consideration of the fact that some immunosuppressants, such as cyclophosphamide, mycophenolate mofetil, metothrexate and leflunomide, are contraindicated in pregnancy and lactation due to their teratogenicity.

REFERENCES

1. Gurevitz SL, Snyder JA, Wessel EK, et al. Systemic lupus erythematosus: A review of the disease and treatment options. *Consult Pharm* 2013 Feb;28(2):110–21. doi:10.4140/TCP.n.2013.110.
2. Tsokos GC. Systemic lupus erythematosus. *N Engl J Med* 2011 Dec;365(22):2110–21. doi:10.1056/NEJMra1100359. PMID 22129255.
3. Giannakopoulos B, Krilis S. The pathogenesis of the antiphospholipid syndrome. *N Engl J Med* 2013 Mar 14;368:1033–44. doi:10.1056/NEJMra1112830.
4. Du VX, Kelchtermans H, de Groot PG, de Laat B. From antibody to clinical phenotype, the black box of the antiphospholipid syndrome: Pathogenic mechanisms of the antiphospholipid syndrome. *Thromb Res* 2013 Aug 2. pii: S0049–3848(13)00326-5. doi:10.1016/j.thromres.2013.07.023. [Epub ahead of print.]
5. Lockshin MD, Kim M, Laskin CA, Guerra M, Branch DW, Merrill J, Petri M, Porter TF, Sammaritano L, Stephenson MD, Buyon J, Salmon JE. Prediction of adverse pregnancy outcome by the presence of lupus anticoagulant, but not anticardiolipin antibody, in patients with antiphospholipid antibodies. *Arthritis Rheum* 2012 Jul;64(7):2311–8. doi:10.1002/art.34402.

6. Kwak-Kim J, Han AR, Gilman-Sachs A, Fishel S, Leong M, Shoham Z. Current trends of reproductive immunology practices in in vitro fertilization (IVF) – a first world survey using IVF-Worldwide.com. *Am J Reprod Immunol* 2013 Jan;69(1):12–20. doi:10.1111/j.1600-0897.2012.01183.x. Epub 2012 Aug 8.

7. Mecacci F, Pieralli A, Bianchi B, Paidas MJ. The impact of autoimmune disorders and adverse pregnancy outcome. *Semin Perinatol* 2007;31:223–6.

8. Bellver J, Pellicer A. Ovarian stimulation for ovulation induction and in vitro fertilization in patients with systemic lupus erythematosus and antiphospholipid syndrome. *Fertil Steril* 2009 Dec;92(6):1803–10.

9. Ostensen M, Clowse M. Pathogenesis of pregnancy complications in systemic lupus erythematosus. *Curr Opin Rheumatol* 2013 Sep;25(5):591–6. doi:10.1097/BOR.0b013e328363ebf7.

10. Lockshin MD. Pregnancy and antiphospholipid syndrome. *Am J Reprod Immunol* 2013 Jun;69(6):585–7. doi:10.1111/aji.12071. Epub 2012 Dec 28.

5

The Patient with Epilepsy

E Campbell and J Craig

CONTENTS

Background

Epilepsy is defined as the condition, or more accurately set of conditions, in which individuals have a tendency to recurrent, usually unprovoked epileptic seizures. It is the most common chronic neurological disorder and affects 4–10 of every 1000 people in the developed world. Women of childbearing age account for 25% of people with epilepsy, and three to four pregnancies in every thousand occur to women with epilepsy.[1] The principles of managing epilepsy are similar for men and women, with antiepileptic drugs (AEDs) the mainstay of treatment. However, epilepsy and the use of AEDs, in particular, have special implications for women of childbearing age.

Women with epilepsy are a high-risk group during pregnancy, and there are many issues to be considered before and during pregnancy to improve the chances of a successful outcome. These include the effects of epilepsy and AEDs on pregnancy, the effects of pregnancy on AEDs and seizure control, and the effects of epilepsy, seizures and, in particular AEDs, on the developing embryo/fetus. Ideally all pregnancies in women with epilepsy should be planned, with optimization of medication regimens and seizure control occurring preconceptually.[2,3]

Impact of Epilepsy and AEDs on IVF

Women with epilepsy appear to have lower rates of childbearing and reduced fertility.[4] The potential reasons include psychological, social and economic factors. Epileptic seizures and interictal epileptiform discharges, particularly with temporal lobe involvement, may disrupt the hypothalamic-pituitary axis by interfering with gonadotrophin-releasing hormone (GnRH) pulsatility.[5] Sexual dysfunction, hormonal and neuroendocrine abnormalities, menstrual disorders, polycystic ovary syndrome (PCOS) and anovulatory cycles have all been reported as more common than in the general population.[6,7] AED treatment may also have an effect on fertility, with abnormal sex hormone levels reported with AEDs which induce the cytochrome P450 system (carbamazepine, phenobarbital, phenytoin, oxcarbazepine, primidone and eslicarbazepine acetate).[8] Links have also been found between sodium valproate and reproductive disorders, in particular PCOS.[9,10] Studies of reproductive function and fertility in men with epilepsy are fewer, but altered testosterone metabolism, hyposexuality, reduced testicular volume, reduced sperm concentration and motility as well as increased incidence of morphologically abnormal sperm have all been reported in association with epilepsy or AEDs.[11]

Impact of Epilepsy and AEDs on Pregnancy

Obstetric Complications

There is conflicting evidence on whether women with epilepsy are at increased risk of obstetric complications during pregnancy. Rates of pregnancy-induced hypertension, pre-eclampsia, pregnancy-related bleeding complications, and caesarean sections do not overall appear to be raised, with more convincing evidence for raised rates of premature contractions and premature labour and delivery and stillbirths and neonatal deaths.[12,13]

The risks of trauma, status epilepticus, or even death from seizures and the psychosocial consequences and restrictions from seizures need to be considered in all women. Figures published from the confidential enquiries into maternal deaths in the UK, covering the period from 1985 to 2008, have repeatedly shown that epilepsy is over-represented as an indirect cause of maternal mortality. The number of maternal deaths occurring in women with epilepsy has increased steadily in each report of the confidential enquiry,[14] from 3 in 1985–1987 to 14 from 2006 to 2008. Considering the prevalence of epilepsy, this represents a 10-fold increased risk of maternal death compared to the background population. Although the exact reasons for the increase are poorly understood, in the most recent report, it was noted that only 6 of the 14 women who died were assessed during pregnancy by someone with expertise in epilepsy.

Fetal Complications

Impact of AEDs

It is accepted that AEDs have an effect on fetal and embryonic development. These include an increased risk for major congenital malformations (MCMs), neurodevelopmental delay and maladaptive behaviours, minor congenital anomalies, to include facial dysmorphism and intra-uterine growth retardation.

Women with epilepsy who are not taking AEDs have a lower risk of MCMs than those who are taking AEDs. Those taking more than one AED are at a greater risk. Overall women with epilepsy who take a single AED in pregnancy have a risk of between 4% and 9% of having an infant with an MCM, that is some two to three times more than the background risk.[15,16]

Not all AEDs have the same risks for MCMs. Valproate, especially in higher doses, has consistently been found to be associated with the highest risk for MCMs.[15,16] Data are available for many other AEDs (Table 5.1) with more reassuring results having been found for carbamazepine,[15,17] lamotrigine[15–18] and levetiracetam.[17,19] For topiramate, MCM rates have been found between those for valproate and other AEDs.[17] From these findings the Food and Drug Administration in the United States has reclassified it a category D drug.

Approximately 30–40% of all patients with epilepsy will be required take more than one AED to achieve the best level of seizure control, for which the risks for MCMs have been considered to be higher.[20] It has been reported that it is when valproate is one of the AEDs used in combination therapy that the risk for MCMs is increased. The North American AED Pregnancy Registry[20] and the International Lamotrigine Pregnancy Registry,[18] respectively, observed MCM rates of 9.1% and 10.7% when lamotrigine was given in a polytherapy regimen with valproate and 2.9% and 2.8% when lamotrigine was given with other AEDs.

TABLE 5.1

Rates of Major Congenital Malformations (MCMs) Following Exposure to Antiepileptic Drug (AED) Monotherapies during Pregnancy

Drug	UK Epilepsy and Pregnancy Register		International Registry of AEDs and Pregnancy (EURAP)		North American AED Pregnancy Registry	
	Number of Exposures	MCM Rate (%)	Number of Exposures	MCM Rate (%)	Number of Exposures	MCM Rate (%)
No AEDs	541	2.4	NA	NA	442	1.1
Carbamazepine	1657	2.6	1402	5.6	1033	3.0
Gabapentin	44[a]	2.3	23	0	145	0.7
Lamotrigine	2098	2.3	1280	2.9	1562	2.0
Levetiracetam	304	0.7	126	1.6	450	2.4
Phenobarbital	11[a]	0	217	7.4	199	5.5
Phenytoin	106[a]	6.6	103	5.8	416	2.9
Topiramate	116[a]	5.2	73	6.8	359	4.2
Valproate	1220	6.7	1010	9.7	323	9.3
Zonisamide	8	0	3	0	90	0

[a] Personal communication. Data to end of December 2012.

Children of women with epilepsy, whether or not they are taking AEDs, are at increased risk of minor anomalies and adverse cognitive outcomes. Specific AED-related fetal syndromes have also been reported for most of the older AEDs, in particular valproate.[21] Maladaptive behaviours and neurodevelopmental disorders have been the subject of more recent study.

With regard to cognitive functioning there is evidence that these vary by AED exposure (Table 5.2), with valproate most often implicated as associated with the worst outcomes.[22–24] A wide range of cognitive deficits, including reduced mean IQ, reduced measures of verbal ability, non-verbal ability, memory and executive function have been reported with valproate exposure, the effects of which may be dose dependent.[24] Two recent studies have also suggested an association between epilepsy, and in particular valproate use, and neurodevelopmental disorders such as Asperger syndrome, attention deficit hyperactivity disorder (ADHD), autistic spectrum disorders and dyspraxia.[25,26] Although further work is required, these results are very concerning. Data for lamotrigine,[23,24] based on a number of studies, are more reassuring as are preliminary data for levetiracetam.[27]

Impact of Seizures

The fetus seems relatively resistant to the effects of seizures, although anecdotal evidence suggests that tonic-clonic seizures may cause fetal bradycardia or miscarriage. More minor seizures (partial, absence or myoclonic) are not felt to be harmful to the fetus. Prospective studies have not shown an association between tonic-clonic seizures and MCMs; however there is evidence that uncontrolled seizures can have an adverse effect on the risks for prematurity and fetal growth,[28] as well as cognitive development.[22]

Impact of IVF and Pregnancy on Epilepsy

Hormonal Effects

Hormonal alterations can affect seizure frequency in women with epilepsy. An increase in seizure frequency around the time of menstruation (catamenial epilepsy) was first clinically documented by Gowers in 1885, but cyclical variations in seizure frequency have been known about since antiquity and were initially attributed to the cycles of the moon.

Experimental evidence from animal studies suggests that changes in seizure frequency during the menstrual cycle may be related to the relative oestrogen and progesterone concentrations, with oestrogens considered to have proconvulsant and progestogens anticonvulsant properties. Human data tend to support this hypothesis, although there appear to be no clear differences in hormonal changes in women with and without catamenial seizures. In human studies, increased seizure frequency has been reported during the follicular phase when oestrogen concentrations are highest. Anovulatory cycles also tend to be associated with higher seizure frequencies, in particular during times of peak oestrogen concentration. Anovulatory cycles tend to be associated with an increase in seizure frequency in the second half of the menstrual cycle, while ovulatory cycles can have one or two peaks in seizure frequency, at around the time of menstruation and/or ovulation.[29]

TABLE 5.2

Effect of Antiepileptic Drug (AED) Exposure during Pregnancy on Neurodevelopment and Rates of Neurodevelopmental Disorders

| | NEAD Study Group, 2013[24] | | Cummings et al., 2011[23] | | Liverpool and Manchester Neurodevelopment Group, 2013[25] | | Christensen et al., 2013[26] | | |
	Number	Mean IQ Age 6 (Mean Difference Compared to Valproate)	Number	Adjusted Odds Ratio for Mild or Significant Developmental Delay (vs. Controls) (95% CI)	Number	Adjusted Odds Ratio of Neurodevelopmental Disorder (vs. Controls) (95% CI)	Number	Adjusted Hazard Ratio of Autistic Spectrum Disorders (vs. Other AEDs) (95% CI)	Adjusted Hazard Ratio of Childhood Autism (vs. Other AEDs) (95% CI)
Valproate	62	97	58	26.1 (4.9–139)	50	6.05 (1.65–24.53)	388	3.0 (1.7–5.4)	4.9 (2.3–10.3)
Lamotrigine	100	108 (+10)	35	1.1 (0.1–13.7)	30	4.06 (0.55–22.20)	647	1.7 (0.8–3.5)	1.7 (0.5–5.2)
Carbamazepine	94	105 (+7)	49	7.7 (1.4–43.1)	50	1.09 (0.06–7.39)	386	1.0 (0.4–2.8)	1.4 (0.4–5.8)
Phenytoin	55	108 (+10)	NA	NA	NA	NA	NA	NA	NA

There are no studies reporting the effect of IVF on seizure frequency. Apart from a few case reports there is little to suggest that IVF treatments cause new-onset seizures or deterioration in seizure control in someone with epilepsy. However, bearing in mind the documented effects of hormonal changes on seizure frequency there is reason to suspect that, at least in some women, the high oestrogen levels resulting from ovarian stimulation during IVF along with the stress associated with the treatment may have a deleterious effect on seizure control.

Seizure Control

Some women will have altered seizure control in pregnancy. It is generally felt that women with well-controlled epilepsy are unlikely to experience a significant change in their seizure frequency. A study of 1956 prospectively identified cases reported that seizure control was unchanged compared to baseline in 63.6%, with 15.9% and 17.3%, respectively, having an improvement and deterioration in seizure control. Of those who entered pregnancy seizure free, 92.7% remained so throughout the entire pregnancy.[30] The reasons for altered control are multiple and include vomiting, stress, altered sleep patterns and problems with compliance.

During pregnancy total serum AED levels may fall with less-marked reductions in non-protein-bound (free) drug concentrations. Many factors contribute, including increased metabolism/excretion, increased plasma volume and reduced protein binding. Total AED concentrations do not predict response during pregnancy, and therefore if serum assessments are to be made measurement of the unbound fraction is the method of choice. This is especially relevant for those AEDs, such as valproate and phenytoin, that are moderately or highly protein bound.

Pronounced alterations in serum levels of lamotrigine have been shown during pregnancy and have been reported as associated with almost 40% of women having a deterioration in seizure control.[31] Falling AED levels have also been found for oxcarbazepine and levetiracetam,[32] although the potential effect on seizure control is less clear. The effect of pregnancy on serum AED levels is summarised in Table 5.3.

TABLE 5.3

Effect of Pregnancy on Total and Free Plasma Levels of Antiepileptic Drugs (AEDs)

AED	Decrease in Total Plasma Concentration (%)	Decrease in Free Concentration (%)
Phenobarbital	55	50
Phenytoin	61	18
Carbamazepine	10–40	4
Valproate	39	25
Lamotrigine	40–60	–
Oxcarbazepine	36–50	–
Levetiracetam	50–60	–

Preparing the Patient with Epilepsy for IVF

Preconceptual Counselling

Preconception counselling should be available for all women with epilepsy, to include those contemplating IVF. While ideally this should start at the time of diagnosis and at subsequent reviews, women of childbearing years with epilepsy do not always recall being given relevant information, and there is a need to repeat this regularly. If a woman with epilepsy is being considered for IVF and does not recall preconception counseling taking place, referral to a preconceptual counseling clinic should be considered before fertility treatment commences. Ideally an organised joint obstetric/neurology preconceptual counseling service should be available, but given the numbers of neurologists and those other specialists with an interest in epilepsy, this is not always possible.

During counselling, re-evaluation of the diagnosis and the need for continued AED medication should take place. Consideration should be given to the type and dose of any AED taken. If it is decided to change from one AED to another it must be emphasized that changeovers can take many months. Since in the changeover period women will be taking two rather than one AED, IVF and pregnancy are best avoided until any changes are complete to avoid the increased risk of MCMs associated with polytherapy regimens.

The risks and benefits of reducing or changing medication should be fully discussed with each individual patient and documentation made of the content of any discussions.

During preconceptual counselling the risks of MCMs and the types of malformations occurring with specific AEDs should be mentioned as should any known risks for cognitive and developmental delay. The genetics of the seizure disorder may also need to be taken into consideration. For example, for autosomal dominant conditions such as tuberous sclerosis there is a 1:2 risk of a child inheriting the condition. Most of the inheritable syndromes which include epilepsy in their phenotype are autosomal recessive, and there is therefore a low risk of children developing the condition. The risk of a child developing epilepsy is dependent on the type of seizure disorder and the number of affected relatives. For generalised epilepsy syndromes there is up to a 10% chance of offspring developing epilepsy, but this is increased if both parents have epilepsy or if the child's siblings develop epilepsy. The risk seems to be lower if only the father has epilepsy compared with if only the mother has epilepsy.

According to guidelines from NICE (National Institute for Health and Care) and SIGN (Scottish Intercollegiate Guidelines Network), all women with epilepsy should take folic acid 5 mg daily before any possibility of pregnancy.[2,3] Although recommended primarily to reduce the risk of MCMs and in particular neural tube defects, there is as yet no evidence that folic acid in any dose reduces the risk of MCMs for AEDs.[33] Data from the Neurodevelopmental Effects of Antiepileptic Drugs (NEAD) study group have demonstrated that periconceptual folic acid positively influenced full-scale IQ in infants exposed to AEDs in utero.[24] Taken alongside results from studies in the general population that have shown a reduced risk of severe language delay with folic acid supplementation in early pregnancy[34] and improved measures of verbal communication with high-dose preconceptual folic acid supplementation,[35] suggests that women with epilepsy should continue high-dose folic acid supplementation throughout pregnancy.

Poor compliance with AED treatment because of nausea or fear of the potential risks from AEDs to the fetus can result in loss of seizure control. Strict adherence to AED regimes should be encouraged throughout IVF and pregnancy.

Management during IVF

Once AED dose and seizure control are optimised, women undertaking IVF treatment should be made aware of the potential influence of ovarian stimulation and the stress of IVF on seizure frequency. Seizure control should be closely monitored during fertility treatment, ideally with regular input from a neurologist or epilepsy specialist, if required. If women experience an increase in seizures during IVF or early pregnancy they should be encouraged to contact their neurologist or epilepsy nurse for advice.

Management in Early Pregnancy

Ideally women with epilepsy should be supervised in an obstetric unit with access to high-resolution ultrasound scanning and the full range of prenatal tests and access to a physician with a specialist interest in epilepsy. Where the last is not available an obstetrician with an interest in medically complicated pregnancies should be identified. The majority of women with epilepsy will have a normal delivery, an unchanged seizure frequency and over a 90% chance of a healthy baby. Considering pregnancies in women with epilepsy are considered high risk careful management by both neurological and obstetric teams is essential.

Abrupt withdrawal or switching of medications during pregnancy should be discouraged due to the potential risks of uncontrolled seizure breakthrough to the mother and baby. The importance of full compliance with AEDs and the need to promote best-possible general health should be stressed.

Women should be encouraged to continue to take high-dose folic acid throughout pregnancy, and in the UK NICE suggests that all pregnant women with epilepsy should be encouraged to notify their pregnancy, or allow their clinician to notify the pregnancy, to the UK Epilepsy and Pregnancy Register.[3]

Management of Labour and the Post-Partum Period

Most women with epilepsy will have a normal uncomplicated vaginal delivery; however, in approximately 2–4% seizures occur during labour or in the following 24 hours. Tonic-clonic seizures may affect fetal oxygenation. Delivery should therefore preferably take place in a unit equipped with facilities for maternal and neonatal resuscitation.

Breastfeeding is to be encouraged. The amount transferred to the infant varies substantially between AEDs. Any concerns that breastfeeding during AED therapy might have a detrimental effect on cognitive development have not been realized. Risk of injury to the infant largely depends on seizure type and frequency. Risks can be minimized if time is allocated to training mothers with epilepsy on safe handling, bathing techniques, feeding, and safe practice around the home.

Key Management Points

1. Women with epilepsy are a high-risk group in pregnancy.
2. All pregnancies to women with epilepsy should be planned with optimisation of AED regimens and seizure control preconceptually.
3. All women with epilepsy should take 5 mg folic acid daily before any possibility of pregnancy.
4. AEDs taken in pregnancy can be associated with adverse fetal outcomes.
5. Overall, rates of MCMs in infants born to women with epilepsy are two to three times higher than the background risk, equating to a risk of between 4% and 9%.
6. The risk of MCMs is higher for those with polytherapy regimens and regimens containing valproate.
7. AEDs, in particular valproate, have been associated with higher risks of neurodevelopmental delay and autistic spectrum disorders.
8. During pregnancy, women with epilepsy should ideally be supervised in a unit with access to high-resolution ultrasound scanning and a physician with a specialist interest in epilepsy or obstetrician with an interest in medically complicated pregnancies.
9. Plasma levels of AEDs may fall during pregnancy and can result in loss of seizure control.
10. There are no studies documenting the effect of IVF on seizure frequency. It is generally felt that women with well-controlled epilepsy are unlikely to experience a significant change in their seizure frequency during pregnancy.

REFERENCES

1. Olafsson E, Hallgrimsson JT, Hauser WA et al. Pregnancies of women with epilepsy: A population-based study in Iceland. *Epilepsia* 1998;39:887–92.
2. Scottish Intercollegiate Guidelines Network. Scottish Intercollegiate Guidelines Network guideline No. 70: diagnosis and management of epilepsy in adults. Issued April 2003, updated October 2005. http://www.sign.ac.uk/guidelines/fulltext/70/.
3. National Institute for Health and Care. National Institute for Health and Care Excellence Clinical Guideline 137: The epilepsies: The diagnosis and management of the epilepsies in adults and children in primary and secondary care. Issued January 2012. http://www.nice.org.uk/cg137.
4. Olafsson E, Hauser WA, Gudmundsson G. Fertility in patients with epilepsy: A population-based study. *Neurology* 1998;51:71–3.
5. Herzog AG, Seibel MM, Schomer DL, Vaitukaitis JL, Geschwind N. Reproductive endocrine disorders in women with partial seizures of temporal lobe origin. *Arch Neurol* 1986;43:341–6.
6. Herzog AG, Coleman AE, Jacobs AR, Klein P, Friedman MN, Drislane FW et al. Interictal EEG discharges, reproductive hormones, and menstrual disorders in epilepsy. *Ann Neurol* 2003;54:625–37.
7. Bilo L, Meo R, Valentino R, DiCarlo C, Striano S, Nappi C. Characterization of reproductive endocrine disorders in women with epilepsy. *J Clin Endocrinol Metab* 2001 Jul;86(7):2950–6.

8. Isojärvi JI, Taubøll E, Herzog AG. Effect of antiepileptic drugs on reproductive endocrine function in individuals with epilepsy. *CNS Drugs* 2005;19(3):207–23.

9. Isojarvi JI, Laatikainen TJ, Pakarinen AJ, Juntunen KT, Myllyla VV. Polycystic ovaries and hyperandrogenism in women taking valproate for epilepsy. *N Engl J Med* 1993;329:1383–8.

10. Morrell MJ, Hayes FJ, Sluss PM, Adams JM, Bhatt M, Ozkara C et al. Hyperandrogenism, ovulatory dysfunction, and polycystic ovary syndrome with valproate versus lamotrigine. *Ann Neurol* 2008;64:200–11.

11. Herzog AG, Drislane FW, Schomer DL, Pennell PB, Bromfield EB, Dworetzky BA et al. Differential effects of antiepileptic drugs on sexual function and hormones in men with epilepsy. *Neurology* 2005;65(7):1016–20.

12. Harden CL, Hopp J, Ting TY et al. Management issues for women with epilepsy – focus on pregnancy (an evidence-based review): I. Obstetrical complications and change in seizure frequency. *Epilepsia* 2009;50:1229–36.

13. Martin PJ, Millac PAH. Pregnancy, epilepsy, management and outcome: A 10 year perspective. *Seizure* 1993;2:277–80.

14. Cantwell R, Clutton-Brock T, Cooper G, Dawson A, Drife J, Garrod D et al. Saving mothers' lives: reviewing maternal deaths to make motherhood safer: 2006–2008. The eighth report of the Confidential Enquiries into Maternal Deaths in the United Kingdom. *BJOG* 2011;118(Suppl 1):1–203.

15. Morrow J, Russell A, Guthrie E et al. Malformation risks of antiepileptic drugs in pregnancy: A prospective study from the UK Epilepsy and Pregnancy Register. *J Neurol Neurosurg Psychiatry* 2006;77:193–8.

16. Tomson T, Battino D, Bonizzoni E, Craig J, Lindhout D, Sabers A et al. EURAP study group. Dose-dependent risk of malformations with antiepileptic drugs: an ananalysis of data from the EURAP epilepsy and pregnancy registry. *Lancet Neurol* 2011;10(7):609–17.

17. Hernández-Díaz S, Smith CR, Shen A, Mittendorf R, Hauser WA, Yerby M et al. North American AED Pregnancy Registry. Comparative safety of antiepileptic drugs during pregnancy. *Neurology* 2012;78(21):1692–9.

18. Cunnington MC, Weil JG, Messenheimer JA, Ferber S, Yerby, M, Tennis P. Final results from 18 years of the International Lamotrigine Pregnancy Registry. *Neurology* 2011;76:1817–23.

19. Mawhinney E, Craig J, Morrow J, Russell A, Smithson WH, Parsons L et al. Levetiracetam in pregnancy: results from the UK and Ireland Epilepsy and Pregnancy Registers. *Neurology* 2013;80:400–5.

20. Holmes LB, Mittendorf R, Shen A, Smith CR, Hernandez-Diaz S. Fetal effects of anticonvulsant polytherapies: different risks from different drug combinations. *Arch Neurol* 2011;68(10):1275–81.

21. Diliberti JH, Farndon PA, Dennis NR, Curry CJR. The fetal valproate syndrome. *Am J Med Genet* 1984;19:473–81.

22. Adab N, Kini U, Vinten J et al. The longer term outcome of children born to mothers with epilepsy. *J Neurol Neurosurg Psychiatry* 2004;75:1575–83.

23. Cummings C, Stewart M, Stevenson M, Morrow J, Nelson J. Neurodevelopment of children exposed in utero to lamotrigine, sodium valproate and carbamazepine. *Arch Dis Child* 2011;96(7):643–7.

24. Meador KJ, Baker GA, Browning N, Cohen MJ, Bromley RL, Clayton-Smith J et al. Fetal antiepileptic drug exposure and cognitive outcomes at age 6 years (NEAD study): A prospective observational study. *Lancet Neurol* 2013;12:244–52.

25. Bromley RL, Mawer GE, Briggs M, Cheyne C, Clayton-Smith J, Garcia-Finana M et al. The prevalence of neurodevelopmental disorders in children prenatally exposed to antiepileptic drugs. *J Neurol Neurosurg Psychiatry* 2013;84(6):637–43.

26. Christensen J, Gronborg TK, Sorensen MJ, Schendel D, Parner ET, Pedersen LH, Vestergaard M. Prenatal valproate exposure and risk of autism spectrum disorders and childhood autism. *JAMA* 2013;309(16):1696–1703.

27. Shallcross R, Bromley RL, Irwin B, Bonnett LJ, Morrow J, Baker GA, on behalf of the Liverpool Manchester Neurodevelopment Group and the UK Epilepsy and Pregnancy Register. Child development following in utero exposure. Levetiracetam vs sodium valproate. *Neurology* 2011;76:383–9.

28. Chen YH, Chiou HY, Lin HC, Lin HL. Effect of seizures during gestation on pregnancy outcomes in women with epilepsy. *Arch Neurol* 2009;66:979–84.

29. Herzog AG, Klein P, Ransil BJ. Three patterns of catamenial epilepsy. *Epilepsia* 1997;38:1082–8.

30. The EURAP Study Group. Seizure control and treatment in pregnancy. Observations from the EURAP Epilepsy Pregnancy Registry. *Neurology* 2006;66(3):354–60.

31. Pennell PB, Newport DJ, Stowe ZN et al. The impact of pregnancy and childbirth on the metabolism of lamotrigine. *Neurology* 2004;62:292–5.

32. Tomson T, Palm R, Källén K, Ben-Menachem E, Söderfeldt B, Danielsson B et al. Pharmacokinetics of levetiracetam during pregnancy, delivery, in the neonatal period, and lactation. *Epilepsia* 2007 Jun;48(6):1111–6.

33. Morrow JI, Hunt SJ, Russell AJ et al. Folic acid use and congenital malformations in offspring of women with epilepsy. A prospective study from the UK Epilepsy and Pregnancy Register. *J Neurol Neurosurg Psychiatry* 2008;80:506–11.

34. Roth C, Magnus P, Schjolberg S, Stoltenberg C, Suren P, McKeague IW et al. Folic acid supplements in pregnancy and severe language delay in children. *JAMA* 2011;306(14):1566–73.

35. Chatzil L, Papadopoulou E, Koutra K, Roumeliotaki T, Georgiou V et al. Effect of high doses of folic acid supplementation in early pregnancy on child neurodevelopment at 18 months of age: The mother-child cohort 'Rhea' study in Crete, Greece. *Public Health Nutr* 2012;15(9):1728–36.

6

The Patient with Inflammatory Bowel Disease

SV Kane and JG Al Hashash

CONTENTS

Background

Over half of the patients diagnosed with inflammatory bowel disease (IBD) are of reproductive age, so being aware of the effect of IBD, be it Crohn's disease or ulcerative colitis, on fertility and fecundity is crucial. Not only can the disease itself interfere with one's ability to conceive, but also several of the medications used for treating these conditions may play a role in altering conception.

Having IBD does not automatically impact an individual's fertility. Patients with ulcerative colitis who have not undergone prior intestinal surgery have comparable fertility rates to patients without ulcerative colitis.[1] Similarly, patients with Crohn's disease who are in remission also have comparable fertility rates to controls with no Crohn's disease.[2] A recent meta-analysis looking at 11 studies demonstrated that patients with ulcerative colitis did not have reduced fertility rates when compared with controls.[3] Although patients with Crohn's disease had some reduction in fertility rates, this was due to voluntary childlessness from fear of bad outcome rather than physiologic involuntary fertility.[3] Active disease, however, is a contributor for decreased fertility in patients with IBD.[4] Patients with active disease tend to have fatigue, anemia, pain, malnutrition, and a diminished quality of life which not only directly affect fertility, but also diminish the desire to conceive. Females with active disease were also noted to have T-cell dysfunction, raising the possibility that an immunologic component may be contributing to the decreased fertility.[5]

Prior surgery, specifically when it involves significant pelvic dissection, such as creation of an ileal pouch anal anastomosis for ulcerative colitis, markedly affects fecundity. This effect is secondary to the scarring and adhesions that form after extensive pelvic dissection leading to tubal obstruction, rather than a direct effect from the underlying IBD. The same outcome of decreased fecundity was noted in patients with familial adenomatous polyposis and no concomitant IBD who underwent ileal pouch anal anastomosis.[6] For this reason, women of reproductive age who are interested in conceiving and who are in need of a total colectomy are advised to undergo a subtotal colectomy with an ileostomy and creation of a Hartmann's pouch (rectal stump) to avoid extensive pelvic dissection, thereby preserving the ability to conceive. A more definitive surgery with pouch creation and ileoanal anastomosis could be considered at a later time once the patient completes childbearing and her family is complete. Other surgical procedures that do not involve extensive pelvic dissection such as creation of an ileorectal anastomosis have not shown such a negative effect on fecundity and fertility rates.[7]

A recent retrospective case-control study looked at the ovarian reserve status of females with Crohn's disease in remission who were of reproductive age.[8] There was no difference in the ovarian reserve between patients with Crohn's disease and those without Crohn's disease in females younger than 30 years of age. However, in patients who were 30 years and older, ovarian reserve was significantly lower in Crohn's disease patients, and this reserve was even further negatively impacted by disease present in the colon. As a consequence of these results, females with Crohn's disease who are interested in childbearing should not delay conception.

Impact of IBD on IVF and Pregnancy

There are no published studies on the direct effect or experience of IBD patients and the success rates of IVF. The emphasis in the literature has been on pregnancy outcomes once conception has occurred. Several population-based studies have demonstrated that females with IBD have more complicated pregnancy outcomes when compared to non-IBD individuals. Stephansson et al. showed an increased risk of moderately preterm birth (between 32 and 36 weeks of gestation), very preterm birth (before 32 weeks of gestation), small-for-gestational-age birth, and caesarean-section (C-section) outcomes in females with Crohn's disease as compared to controls.[9] In a separate population-based study, the same group evaluated females with ulcerative colitis and showed that the risks of moderately preterm birth, very preterm birth, small-for-gestational-age birth, C-section, and preterm deaths were significantly higher in patients with ulcerative colitis when compared to controls.[10] Mahadevan et al. concluded that spontaneous abortion rates, eclampsia/preeclampsia, abruption placenta, placenta previa, and prolonged/premature rupture of membranes were more common in IBD patients.[11] Bortoli et al. recently published results on a prospective study that showed no difference between IBD patients and non-IBD patients with regards to preterm deliveries, C-sections, birth weights, and abortions.[12] It is important to mention that the majority of IBD patients in this particular study were in remission at time of conception and remained in remission throughout the pregnancy.

Molnar et al. conducted a case-control study comparing pregnancy outcomes in the same patients before and after their diagnosis with IBD.[13] The investigators demonstrated that preterm birth and low birth weight were more common in women after their diagnosis with IBD. Subgroup analysis of ulcerative colitis patients alone showed significantly higher preterm births in these women after their diagnosis of ulcerative colitis. Location and extent of disease, presence of perianal complications, and type of delivery did not impact pregnancy outcomes.

Whether congenital anomalies are more common in women affected by IBD remains controversial. Dominitz et al. compared pregnancy outcomes between IBD patients and controls.[14] Results showed that patients with Crohn's disease had significantly worse pregnancy outcomes in terms of preterm delivery, low birth weight, and small-for-gestational-age infants when compared to controls. Although women with ulcerative colitis were not found to have higher rates of preterm delivery or low-birth-weight children, these women were noted to have an increased risk of having a child with congenital anomalies as compared to women who were controls. Cornish et al. conducted a meta-analysis, and the results pertaining to congenital anomalies were predominantly driven by the Dominitz et al. study and showed an increased risk of congenital abnormalities in children born to women affected by IBD (odds ratio [OR] 2.37; 95% confidence interval [CI] 1.47–3.82); subgroup analysis showed that the increased risk was seen only in ulcerative colitis patients and not in those with Crohn's disease.[15]

Active disease at the time of conception and during gestation has been shown to lead to worse pregnancy outcomes, although some other studies failed to show this association. Active disease at the time of conception was associated with increased risk for fetal loss and preterm birth, while active disease during pregnancy was associated with increased risk of preterm birth and low birth weight.[16–18] Mahadevan et al.'s northern California study, however, failed to show an association between disease activity and worse pregnancy outcomes.[11] This may have been because many of the recruited patients were in remission at the time of recruitment to the study. Similarly, Molnar et al. did not show an association between disease activity and worse pregnancy outcomes.[13] Interestingly, though, children born to mothers with active ulcerative colitis during pregnancy were found to have increased risk of childhood diseases.

Impact of IVF and Pregnancy on IBD

In patients with controlled disease activity, pregnancy has not been shown to increase the risk for an IBD flare. Rates for IBD flares are comparable in pregnant women and non-pregnant controls. Nielson et al. demonstrated that the relapse rates of ulcerative colitis and Crohn's disease in pregnant women were similar to the rates seen in non-pregnant women.[17,18] Particularly, relapse rates for pregnant women with ulcerative colitis were 34% per year as compared to 32% for non-pregnant women.[17] When women conceive while their disease is in remission, up to 80% of women remain in remission throughout the pregnancy.[19]

Pederson et al. recently conducted a prospective study on IBD activity in pregnant women compared to age-matched, disease location and disease activity-matched non-pregnant women.[20] Data were collected during each trimester and at 6 months postpartum. Of the Crohn's disease patients who conceived while in remission, the relapse rate whether pregnant or not was similar. Of the Crohn's patients who conceived while their disease was active, over 50% continued to have active disease during their pregnancy, which is higher than the 33% of non-pregnant Crohn's patients. Different from Crohn's disease, ulcerative colitis patients who conceived while in remission were at a higher risk to develop active disease during their pregnancy when compared to non-pregnant controls (HR 2.74; 95% CI 1.61–4.65). The flares were more common during the first two trimesters and in the first 3 months postpartum. To date, the only possible explanation as to why ulcerative colitis is more unstable than Crohn's disease in pregnancy is the shift in the immune environment that occurs as a consequence of maternal response to the fetus.[21]

Women who conceive while their disease is active greatly influence their disease activity and course during pregnancy. Miller concluded that 45% of women with ulcerative colitis who conceive with active disease tend to have a worsening flare during pregnancy, while 24% will have stable active disease.[22] The remainder of the patients experienced resolution of their flare. Among Crohn's disease patients who conceived during active disease, a third of the patients had stable active disease, a third had worsening disease, and a third achieved remission.[22]

Preparing the IBD Patient for IVF

Again, the data on IVF specific to IBD is very scarce. The main target for any woman before pregnancy is to achieve adequate control of her disease prior to conception. This includes discontinuation of medications such as methotrexate and thalidomide, medications used to treat certain patients with active Crohn's disease. Methotrexate should be discontinued up to at least 6 months prior to conception because it may persist in tissues for long periods.[23] Thalidomide should be discontinued at least 1 month prior to conception.[24]

Recurrent spontaneous abortion is a category of infertility. Almost half of these abortions are a consequence of chromosomal abnormalities in the embryo. Other causes are attributed to inflammation at the implantation site which leads to embryo rejection. Increased production of Th1 cytokines such as tumor necrosis factor (TNF) α has been linked to recurrent abortions and infertility. For this, normalization of TNFα has been proposed as a possible approach for some of the cases of infertility, specifically the ones related to overproduction of the Th1 response. In 2008, through a retrospective study, Winger and Reed showed that the addition of either intravenous immunoglobulin alone or immunoglobulin and anti-TNF therapy to standard anti-coagulation increased the rates of live births in women with recurrent spontaneous abortions.[25] The same group published a follow-up study the next year investigating whether treatment with adalimumab and/or intravenous immunoglobulin increased IVF success rates among young women with infertility due to an elevated Th1/Th2.[5] This study concluded that both adalimumab and intravenous immunoglobulin therapy improved IVF rates in these patients.[5] Adalimumab has shown to be an effective drug at treating certain patients with infertility and recurrent abortions.[26] While the efficacy of these therapies remains to be confirmed in prospective randomized trials, the clinical ramifications of these studies suggest that anti-TNF agents not be stopped prior to planned IVF procedures.

Management of IBD during IVF Treatment

As mentioned, it is critical to achieve remission prior to attempting IVF treatment. Active disease has been shown to lead to poor pregnancy outcomes, and active disease itself may worsen during the pregnancy, requiring more aggressive medical and at times surgical interventions. This translates to the clinical recommendation that women continue on their current IBD regimen to maintain disease remission. There are no reports of any increased complication risk for oocyte retrieval in patients with IBD. The use of prophylactic antibiotics should be at the discretion of the gynecologist, but most gastroenterologists would suggest that unless absolutely necessary patients avoid the use of antibiotics as some can cause a flare of disease.

Management of IBD in Early Pregnancy

Most women aim at discontinuing all their medications, whether IBD related or not, prior to conception because of fear of potential side effects on the fetus. Despite studies that continue to support the safety of using most IBD medications during pregnancy, patients and at times their physicians feel uncomfortable continuing these medications. Unless a woman is taking methotrexate or thalidomide, physicians should encourage their patients to continue their maintenance IBD medications during pregnancy. Achieving and maintaining disease remission should be the goal in managing pregnant patients in order to decrease the rates of complications and poor outcome for both mother and child.

Mesalamine products have shown to be safe in pregnancy. Although mesalamine and its metabolite are found in cord plasma, there have not been increased fetal abnormalities associated with the use of these drugs at 2–3 grams daily.[27] Despite early reports that suggested teratogenecity with sulfasalazine, larger studies showed that sulfasalazine is considered safe in pregnancy. Sulfasalazine crosses the placenta but has not been associated with any fetal abnormalities. Due to sulfasalazine's potential anti-folate effects, it is important to supplement women receiving sulfasalazine with 1 mg of folic acid twice daily in the prenatal and perinatal periods to avoid fetal neural tube defects. Sulfasalazine and the mesalamine agents, with the exception of olsalazine, Asacol and Asacol HD, are considered Category B in pregnancy. The last three drugs are considered Category C. Asacol has recently been discontinued and no longer is available. Asacol HD, however, remains on the market and is a C due to its dibutyl pthalate in the capsule coating. At mega-doses of dibutyl pthalate (at least 190 times the dose used for the Asacol HD coating), this drug has showed external and skeletal malformations as well as effects on the male reproductive system in animal studies.

Immunomodulators in the form of 6-mercaptopurine and its prodrug, azthioprine, are widely used in IBD. Although they are classified as Category D drugs in pregnancy, the recommendation is to continue these medications during pregnancy in order to maintain disease remission. Animal studies showed increased teratogenecity with the use of these drugs, but the doses utilized in the animal studies were much higher than the doses used in humans for treatment of IBD. Moreover, in the animal studies, the immunomodulators were given intravenously and through the intraperi-toneum rather than through the oral route as is prescribed for IBD patients. Studies from the transplant literature in addition to others following IBD patients, including the study from the Cancers Et Surrisque Associe aux Maladies inflammatoires intes-tinales en France (CESAME) study group, support the use of thiopurines in pregnant women.[28]

Methotrexate is a Category X drug in pregnancy. It should not be used in women who plan on becoming pregnant up to at least 6 months before attempting conception. Methotrexate is teratogenic, and its use in the first trimester greatly interferes with organogenesis and leads to multiple congenital anomalies. Women of childbearing potential are asked to be on at least one form, preferably two forms, of contraception while on the methotrexate. Methotrexate embryopathy, a syndrome associated with the use of methotrexate, is characterized by limb abnormalities, small low-set ears, micrognathia, intrauterine growth retardation, hypoplastic supraorbital ridges, and at times mental retardation. Methotrexate takes a longer time to clear from the tissue, so the drug needs to be stopped at least 6 months before conception.

Anti-TNF therapy includes infliximab, adalimumab, and certolizumab, and all are considered Category B drugs in pregnancy and are generally safe for use dur-ing pregnancy. Natalizumab on the other hand is a Category C drug. Infliximab is an immunoglobulin (Ig) G1 antibody that has been shown to cross the placenta after week 20 of gestation. For this reason, it is safe to be used in the first two trimesters and does not intervene with organogenesis. Due to the immaturity of the reticuloendethelial systems of infants and their inability to clear antibody, infliximab is detectable in the bloodstreams of newborns for a few months after birth. Pediatricians need to be aware of this to avoid vaccinating these infants with live vaccines until they are older than 6 months of age. Results from the Crohn's Therapy, Resource, Evaluation and Assessment Tool (TREAT) Registry, a prospective registry for Crohn's disease patients, failed to show increased rates of fetal malformations, miscarriage, or neonatal complications in patients who received infliximab compared to those who were infliximab naive.[29] Similar to inf-liximab, adalimumab is an IgG1 antibody that also crosses the placenta after week 20 and is present in the bloodstreams of newborns until 6 months of age. Studies have shown that the use of adalimumab in pregnant patients does not increase the rates of spontaneous abortion, stillbirth, congenital malformation, and preterm delivery when compared to the rates from the general population.[23,30] Although there are no guidelines, it is generally recommended to administer the last dose of infliximab or adalimumab 6–8 weeks prior to the estimated delivery date in attempts to minimize placental transfer to the fetus.[31,32] Certolizumab pegol is a pegylated Fab' fragment of humanized anti-TNFα monoclonal antibody. This mol-ecule is not actively transported across the placenta and thus is safe to continue throughout pregnancy. Natalizumab is an IgG4 molecule that targets the adhesion molecule α4-integrin. To date, there is very limited data regarding the use of this medication in pregnancy. The natalizumab global safety database review showed no increase in birth defects among newborns whose mothers were treated with natalizumab during their pregnancy.[33]

Corticosteroids are considered a Category C medication during pregnancy. There have been studies reporting orofacial cleft defects in infants born to mothers who have received corticosteroids during their first trimester of pregnancy. A larger prospective study refuted these findings and showed no increased rates of orofacial cleft defects in these infants. Transplant literature linked steroid use to adrenal insufficiency in both the newborn and the mother as well as premature rupture of membranes.

Key Management Points

1. Active disease is a contributor for decreased fertility in patients with IBD. It is very important to maintain disease remission pre-conception and throughout pregnancy.
2. Pelvic dissection surgery as is done with creation of an ileal pouch anal anastomosis markedly affects fecundity.
3. Although still controversial, active disease at time of conception and during gestation has been shown to lead to worse pregnancy outcomes.
4. Rates for IBD flares are comparable in pregnant women and non-pregnant controls.
5. All IBD medications except for thalidomide and methotrexate can be continued in patients who are planning on conceiving and pregnant patients.

REFERENCES

1. Willoughby CP, Truelove SC. Ulcerative colitis and pregnancy. *Gut* 1980;21:469–474.
2. Khosla R, Willoughby CP, Jewell DP. Crohn's disease and pregnancy. *Gut* 1984; 25:52–56.
3. Tavernier N, Fumery M, Peyrin-Biroulet L, et al. Systematic review: fertility in non-surgically treated inflammatory bowel disease. *Aliment Pharmacol Ther* 2013; 38(8):847–853.
4. Hudson M, Flett G, Sinclair TS, et al. Fertility and pregnancy in inflammatory bowel disease. *Int J Gynaecol Obstet* 1997;58(2):229–237.
5. Winger EE, Reed JL, Ashoush S, et al. Treatment with adalimumab (Humira) and intravenous immunoglobulin improves pregnancy rates in women undergoing IVF. *Am J Reprod Immunol* 2009;61(2):113–120.
6. Olsen KO, Juul S, Bulow S, et al. Female fecundity before and after operation for familial adenomatous polyposis. *Br J Surg* 2003;90:227–231.
7. Mortier PE, Gambiez L, Karoui M, et al. Colectomy with ileorectal anastomosis preserves female fertility in ulcerative colitis. *Gastroenterol Clin Biol* 2006;30(4): 594–597.
8. Freour T, Miossec C, Bach-Ngohou K. Ovarian reserve in young women of reproductive age with Crohn's disease. *Inflamm Bowel Dis* 2012;18(8): 1515–1522.
9. Stephansson O, Larsson H, Pedersen L, et al. Crohn's disease is a risk factor for preterm birth. *Clin Gastroenterol Hepatol* 2010;8(6):509–515.
10. Stephansson O, Larsson H, Pedersen L, et al. Congenital abnormalities and other birth outcomes in children born to women with ulcerative colitis in Denmark and Sweden. *Inflamm Bowel Dis* 2011;17(3):795–801.
11. Mahadevan U, Sandborn WJ, Li DK, et al. Pregnancy outcomes in women with inflammatory bowel disease: A large community based study from Northern California. *Gastroenterology* 2007;133(4):1106–1112.

12. Bortoli A, Pedersen N, Duricova D, et al. Pregnancy outcome in inflammatory bowel disease: prospective European case-control ECCO-EpiCom study, 2003–2006. *Aliment Pharmacol Ther* 2011;34(7):724–734.

13. Molnar T, Farkas K, Nagy F, et al. Pregnancy outcome in patients with inflammatory bowel disease according to the activity of the disease and the medical treatment: A case-control study. *Scand J Gastroenterol* 2010;45(11):1302–1306.

14. Dominitz JA, Young JC, Boyko EJ. Outcomes of infants born to mothers with inflammatory bowel disease: A population-based cohort study. *Am J Gastroenterol* 2002;97(3):641–648.

15. Cornish J, Tan E, Teare J, et al. A meta-analysis on the influence of inflammatory bowel disease on pregnancy. *Gut* 2007;56(6):830–837.

16. Morales M, Berney T, Jenny A, et al. Crohn's disease as a risk factor for the outcome of pregnancy. *Hepatogastroenterology* 2000;47(36):1595–1598.

17. Nielson OH, Andreasson B, Bondesen S, et al. Pregnancy in ulcerative colitis. *Scand J Gastroenterol* 1983;18(6):735–742.

18. Nielson OH, Andreasson B, Bondesen S. Pregnancy in Crohn's disease. *Scand J Gastroenterol* 1984;19(6):724–732.

19. Mogadam M, Korelitz BI, Ahmed SW, et al. The course of inflammatory bowel disease during pregnancy and postpartum. *Am J Gastroenterol* 1981;75:265–269.

20. Pederson N, Bortoli A, Duricova D, et al. The course of inflammatory bowel disease during pregnancy and postpartum: A prospective European ECCO-EpiCom study of 209 pregnant women. *Aliment Pharmacol Ther* 2013;38(5):501–512.

21. Sykes L, MacIntyre DA, Yap XJ, et al. Changes in the Th1:Th2 cytokine bias in pregnancy and the effects of the anti-inflammatory cyclopentenone prostaglandin 15-deoxy-(12,14)-prostaglandin J2. *Mediators Inflamm* 2012;2012:416739.

22. Miller JP. Inflammatory bowel disease in pregnancy: A review. *J R Soc Med* 1986;79(4):221–225.

23. Dubinsky M, Abraham B, Mahadevan U. Management of the pregnant IBD patient. *Inflamm Bowel Dis* 2008;14(12):1736–1750.

24. Calgene Corporation. Thalomid. Product information 2000. Calgene Corporation, Summit, NJ.

25. Winger EE, Reed JL. Treatment with tumor necrosis factor inhibitors and intravenous immunoglobulin improves live birth rates in women with recurrent spontaneous abortion. *Am J Reprod Immunol* 2008;60:8–16.

26. Clark DA. Anti-TNFα therapy in immune-mediated subfertility: State of the art. *J Reprod Immunol* 2010;85:15–24.

27. Rahimi R, Nifkar S, Rezaie A, et al. Pregnancy outcome in women with inflammatory bowel disease following exposure to 5-aminosalicylic acid drugs: A meta-analysis. *Reprod Toxicol* 2008;25(2):271–275.

28. Coelho J, Beaugerie L, Colombel JF, et al. Pregnancy outcome in patients with inflammatory bowel disease treated with thiopurines: Cohort from the CESAME Study. *Gut* 2011;60(2):198–203.

29. Lichenstein GR, Feagan BG, Cohen RD, et al. Serious infections and mortality in association with therapies for Crohn's disease: TREAT registry. *Clin Gastroenterol Hepatol* 2006;4:621–630.

30. Norgard B, Hundborg HH, Jacobsen BA, et al. Disease activity in pregnant women with Crohn's disease and birth outcomes: A regional Danish cohort study. *Am J Gastroenterol* 2007;102(9):1947–1954.

31. Ng SW, Mahadevan U. Management of inflammatory bowel disease in pregnancy. *Expert Rev Clin Immunol* 2013;9(2):161–174.

32. Moscandrew M, Kane SV. Inflammatory bowel diseases and management considerations: Fertility and pregnancy. *Curr Gastroenterol Rep* 2009;11(5):395–399.
33. Nazareth M, Hogge GS, Cristiano L, et al. Natalizumab use during pregnancy. Presented at: Annual meeting of the American College of Gastroenterology. Orlando, FL, USA, October 3–8, 2008.

7

The Patient with Hypertension

BB van Rijn and MA Coleman

CONTENTS

Introduction

Chronic hypertension currently affects 1–3% of women of childbearing age, and this figure is likely to show an upward trend due to increasing maternal age and rising obesity rates.[1,2] Common conditions leading to impaired fertility (e.g. polycystic ovary syndrome [PCOS], premature ovarian failure, advanced maternal age and obesity) are all associated with above-average rates of chronic hypertension. In women eligible for IVF, pre-existent hypertension has implications for pregnancy outcome, as well as risks for long-term maternal and fetal health.[3] Management of hypertension in patients undergoing IVF is further challenged by safety concerns for the developing foetus, as some drugs are teratogenic or contraindicated in pregnancy, and antihypertensive treatment may affect fetal growth.

Impact of Hypertension on IVF Outcomes

Risks of hypertension in IVF patients are mainly related to its association with an increased incidence of hypertensive disorders in pregnancy.[4] There is no evidence to suggest that hypertension directly affects the success rate of IVF in terms of ongoing pregnancy rates or incidence of first-trimester pregnancy loss.[5] However, patients who undergo IVF are generally older and primiparous, which can affect the prevalence of chronic hypertension, as well as the risk of obstetric complications.[6]

There are three types of hypertension in pregnancy: (1) chronic hypertension, which is defined as a blood pressure greater than 140/90 mm Hg that either pre-dates pregnancy or develops before 20 weeks gestational age; (2) pregnancy-induced hypertension, which develops after 20 weeks gestational age; and (3) preeclampsia, which is defined by pregnancy-induced hypertension associated with proteinuria. Most of the morbidity is concentrated among pregnancies that are complicated by preeclampsia, which affects about 2% of all pregnancies. The risk of preeclampsia after IVF is reported to be higher than in the general population,[7] although data on the actual prevalence are lacking, and the risk is likely to be variable and dependent on the presence of pre-existing conditions (including chronic hypertension, obesity and PCOS) and the number of twin pregnancies.[8]

Further, women with pre-existent hypertension are at risk of abnormal placental development that not only predisposes to preeclampsia, but also increases the risk of stillbirth, placental abruption and fetal growth restriction.[9] Consequently, hypertensive women are more likely to require preterm delivery, which is reflected in higher perinatal mortality rates in women with prepregnancy chronic hypertension.[10] A large cohort study from South Australia indicated that assisted reproductive technology is itself an independent risk factor for perinatal mortality with an odds ratio of 3.16 after adjustment for other maternal risk factors.[11] However, it is unclear to what extent this risk resides in the need for assisted conception or the treatment itself, as no matched sibling data are yet available.[12,13]

How placental development is affected by hypertension is unclear, but recent data suggest that hypertension has a negative impact on trophoblast invasion and spiral artery remodelling leading to abnormal development of the placental bed.[14] It is unclear if IVF treatment itself increases the risk of placental disorders even further. Adverse obstetric outcomes related to poor placental development, including small-for-gestational age infants, placental abruption and hypertensive disorders of pregnancy, occur more often after IVF compared to the general population,[8,15] but similar increases have been found for subfertile women who conceive without assisted reproductive technology.[16]

Patients undergoing IVF treatment with oocyte donation are more likely to have chronic hypertension and more often develop pregnancy-induced hypertension than patients undergoing regular IVF. This could be related to the advanced maternal age and higher prevalence of other pre-existent risk factors in women accepting egg donation, although it has been suggested that this effect may have an immunological basis.[17] Twin pregnancies further increase the risk of gestational hypertension, preeclampsia and preterm birth. In patients with chronic hypertension, single-embryo transfer is recommended to reduce the risk of blood pressure-related adverse pregnancy outcomes in twins.[18]

Impact of IVF on Hypertension

There is no evidence to suggest that IVF treatment, or pregnancy resulting from IVF, worsens pre-existing hypertension in the long term. However, in patients with hypertension secondary to renal disease, pregnancy may aggravate renal dysfunction with potential irreversible loss of kidney function. This is particularly true for women who develop superimposed preeclampsia, although the effect sizes are uncertain. During IVF treatment, blood pressure may show a mild increase at hospital visits (e.g. at oocyte pickup or embryo transfer), similar to other types of 'white coat' hypertension, and blood pressure measurements before and after treatment are recommended.

Preparing the Patient for IVF

Before commencing IVF treatment, it is important to identify the cause of hypertension and especially to exclude any secondary causes, as they are often serious diseases and can potentially become life threatening in pregnancy. Table 7.1 provides an overview of potential underlying conditions that cause chronic hypertension. The commonest secondary causes of hypertension in patients of childbearing age are renal and cardiac diseases, in particular patients with renal disease as a result of reflux nephropathy, renal artery stenosis or glomerulonephritis. Other conditions that may be found are endocrine disorders, such as Cushing's syndrome and phaeochromocytoma. If a patient has been previously investigated appropriately and it can reasonably be assumed that she has essential hypertension, there is no need to repeat these investigations prior to IVF treatment. However, in all patients presenting with hypertension it is advisable to take a detailed history that includes questions related to potential secondary causes and to repeat any tests if needed. It is also advisable to perform a single urinalysis in all women, including those with essential hypertension, to identify proteinuria and haematuria as possible indicators of renal or vascular damage, as well as glycosuria as a potential marker of underlying diabetes mellitus.

For women with hypertension that is newly diagnosed, hypertension that is not associated with a positive family history, hypertension that is discovered before the age of 30 years or hypertension that has not been investigated previously, thorough investigations are warranted prior to IVF treatment. To investigate secondary causes, physical examinations should include palpation of the femoral pulses to exclude radiofemoral delay associated with aortic coarctation, auscultation to identify heart murmurs and renal bruits suggestive of renal artery stenosis and inspection of any features of Cushing's syndrome. Relevant laboratory investigations are a simple serum creatinine, urea and electrolytes screen to exclude renal impairment

TABLE 7.1

Secondary Causes of Chronic Hypertension

Renal disease
Reflux nephropathy
Chronic kidney disease
Glomerulonephritis
Adult polycystic kidney disease
Renovascular hypertension

Cardiac disease
Aortic coarctation

Endocrine disorders
Conn's syndrome
Cushing's syndrome
Phaeochromocytoma
Hyperparathyroidism

Drug induced or drug related
Cocaine

and hypokalaemia, liver function tests and assessment of calcium status to exclude hypercalcaemia. In patients with symptoms suggestive of phaeochromocytoma (palpitations, labile hypertension, flushes) urinary catecholamines should be measured. Renal ultrasound examination can be useful to exclude renal scarring and hydronephrosis, polycystic kidney disease (especially in those patients with a positive family history that suggests an autosomal dominant inheritance pattern) and small kidneys in chronic renal failure. Adrenal tumours (e.g. found in Conn's syndrome) may be detected by abdominal ultrasound scanning.

Further, counselling of hypertensive patients prior to IVF should take into account any relevant co-morbidities and additional risk factors that may potentiate the risk of adverse pregnancy outcomes (e.g. obesity, diabetes, smoking, renal and cardiac disease). For example, the risk of superimposed preeclampsia in patients with chronic hypertension is substantially higher in obese women with diabetes, compared to non-diabetic patients with normal body mass index. Women with renal impairment should be aware of the potential risks of aggravating their renal disease in pregnancy with possible irreversible kidney damage and loss of renal function, although this has not been investigated thoroughly. Careful considerations should also be made when patients appear to have hypertension secondary to a hereditary condition (e.g. polycystic kidney disease), where genetic counselling and prenatal screening may be appropriate.

Antihypertensive Medication

Patients should be advised to change their antihypertensive medication to preparations that can safely be used in pregnancy (Table 7.2). First-choice antihypertensive drugs are either beta-blockers or alpha receptor agonists. Calcium antagonists (e.g. the calcium channel blocker nifedipine) are also frequently used, although less information is available on safety. Angiotensin-converting enzyme (ACE) inhibitors should be avoided, as they have been shown to potentially cause damage to the fetal kidney with associated renal failure and neonatal mortality.[19,20] Diuretics are also contraindicated because of their presumed negative effect on placental blood flow, although accurate

TABLE 7.2

Antihypertensive Medication for Preconceptional Treatment of Chronic Hypertension

First choice	
Labetalol	Safe to use
Methyldopa	Safe to use
Second choice	
Nifedipine	Safe to use
Other types	
Beta-blockers (e.g. atenolol, bisoprolol)	Safe to use, but limited data on efficacy and fetal risks
Calcium antagonists (e.g. amlodipine)	Safe to use, but limited data on efficacy and fetal risks
ACE inhibitors (e.g. enalapril, ramipril, lisinopril)	Contraindicated, associated with renal failure, teratogenicity and infant mortality
Angiotensin receptor blockers (e.g. losartan)	Contraindicated, associated with placental dysfunction
Diuretics (e.g. thiazide, furosemide)	Contraindicated, associated with placental dysfunction

studies are lacking.[21] The most commonly prescribed types of medication are labetalol and methyldopa which are generally considered to be equally safe.[1,21] Optimal blood pressure control is uncertain and is currently the subject of a large randomized trial evaluating different target blood pressure ranges.[22] Most likely, optimal blood pressure control is achieved when diastolic blood pressure is maintained between 70 and 90 mm Hg and systolic blood pressure is maintained between 120 and 140 mm Hg. Notably, antihypertensive treatment in pregnancy does not reduce the incidence of preeclampsia and does not appear to improve pregnancy outcome.[21] Antihypertensive treatment should therefore primarily be aimed at protecting patients against severe or malignant hypertension, and treatment of mild-to-moderate hypertension (systolic blood pressure 140–160 mm Hg and diastolic blood pressure 90–110 mm Hg) probably has no proven benefit.[23] Some studies have found an association between the use of labetalol and a reduction in infants' birth weight. However, this was not confirmed by others and may have been attributable to the antihypertensive-induced fall in blood pressure rather than to the specific medication type.[21]

Managing the IVF Cycle

Patients with chronic hypertension should have blood pressure monitoring before, during and after IVF treatment, and secondary causes of hypertension and relevant co-morbidities (e.g. diabetes mellitus and obesity) should be treated and monitored accordingly. There are no studies that suggest that chronic hypertension is associated with the prevalence of ovarian hyperstimulation syndrome (OHSS) or is aggravated by ovarian stimulation or IVF treatment. Some studies have reported a higher incidence of pregnancy-induced hypertension after OHSS,[7,24] but this was not found by others.[25] Equally, poor responders are not more likely to develop gestational hypertension.[26]

Aspirin supplementation has been shown to reduce the risk of preeclampsia in patients with a high a priori risk (e.g. a previous episode of severe preeclampsia), but large randomized trials do not support routine use of aspirin in pregnant women on the basis of chronic hypertension alone.[27] Also, based on a recent meta-analysis, preconceptional aspirin use in IVF patients did not reduce the risk of hypertensive pregnancy complications or preterm delivery.[28] Taken together, routine aspirin use in hypertensive patients undergoing IVF should not currently be recommended.

Other types of prophylactic agents to prevent preeclampsia are less well studied in IVF patients and have only been tested when initiated in the first or second trimester of pregnancy. A recent meta-analysis of 12 studies including more than 15,000 women showed that supplementation with calcium (1.5 g/day) during pregnancy lowered blood pressure and reduced the risk of preeclampsia (relative risk 0.48, 95% confidence interval [CI] 0.33–0.69).[29] The effect was greatest for women at high risk and with low calcium intake. However, there are no data on preconceptional prescription of calcium supplements, or on calcium supplementation prior to IVF treatment, making its safety and efficacy in IVF patients questionable.

Antioxidants (including vitamin C and E supplementation) do not reduce hypertensive complications of pregnancy and do not improve pregnancy outcome.[30] Preconceptional folic acid supplementation should be recommended in all women undergoing IVF to prevent neural tube defects, similar to the advice given to women who conceive spontaneously.

Post-IVF Follow-Up

There is a well-established link between hypertensive complications of pregnancy and long-term maternal risk of hypertension, coronary artery disease, stroke and other cardiovascular diseases.[31,32] It is not clear whether preconceptional cardiovascular risk changes after IVF, after pregnancy, or after pregnancy-associated hypertensive complications (e.g. preeclampsia). Most likely, pre-existent chronic hypertension will remain after delivery and thus requires monitoring and regular cardiovascular risk assessment postpartum.[33,34]

There is increasing evidence that periconceptional cardiovascular health of the mother has potential long-term implications for fetal growth and development.[12] In particular, infants with a low birth weight more commonly develop metabolic syndrome, diabetes and cardiovascular disease in adulthood.[35] Infants who do not achieve their growth potential due to an adverse environment (e.g. hypertension and metabolic changes) around the time of conception and early placentation may show adaptive changes at critical stages of fetal development that increase their later-life susceptibility to metabolic and cardiovascular diseases. This so-called developmental origins of health and disease (DOHaD) effect has now been demonstrated in various populations and across the spectrum of normal to low birth weight. As yet, the impact of pre-existent chronic hypertension on long-term cardiovascular outcomes in children born to mothers after IVF treatment has not been established.[12] Also, the implications of preconceptional antihypertensive treatment on fetal development and long-term health are unknown and warrant further research.

Summary of Management Options

1. Excluding secondary causes of hypertension
2. Counselling about the increased risk of preeclampsia, fetal growth restriction and other adverse pregnancy outcomes in women with hypertension prior to IVF treatment
3. Optimizing blood pressure control prior to pregnancy with antihypertensive drugs considered safe in pregnancy with beta-blockers or methyldopa first-choice drugs
4. Creating awareness of the potential long-term cardiovascular risks for mothers and children affected by hypertensive disorders of pregnancy and poor fetal growth

REFERENCES

1. Bateman BT, Hernandez-Diaz S, Huybrechts KF, Palmsten K, Mogun H, Ecker JL, Fischer MA. Patterns of outpatient antihypertensive medication use during pregnancy in a Medicaid population. *Hypertension.* 2012;60:913–920.
2. Kuklina EV, Ayala C, Callaghan WM. Hypertensive disorders and severe obstetric morbidity in the United States. *Obstetrics and Gynecology.* 2009;113:1299–1306.
3. Ombelet W, Cadron I, Gerris J, De Sutter P, Bosmans E, Martens G, Ruyssinck G, Defoort P, Molenberghs G, Gyselaers W. Obstetric and perinatal outcome of 1655

ICSI and 3974 IVF singleton and 1102 ICSI and 2901 IVF twin births: A comparative analysis. *Reproductive Biomedicine Online*. 2005;11:76–85.

4. Roberts CL, Algert CS, Morris JM, Ford JB, Henderson-Smart DJ. Hypertensive disorders in pregnancy: A population-based study. *The Medical Journal of Australia*. 2005;182:332–335.

5. Kharazmi E, Dossus L, Rohrmann S, Kaaks R. Pregnancy loss and risk of cardio-vascular disease: A prospective population-based cohort study (EPIC-Heidelberg). *Heart*. 2011;97:49–54.

6. Reproductive Endocrinology and Infertility Committee, Family Physicians Advisory Committee, Maternal-Fetal Medicine Committee, Executive and Council of the Society of Obstetricians, Liu K, Case A. Advanced reproductive age and fertility. *Journal of Obstetrics and Gynaecology Canada*. 2011;33: 1165–1175.

7. Courbiere B, Oborski V, Braunstein D, Desparoir A, Noizet A, Gamerre M. Obstetric outcome of women with *in vitro* fertilization pregnancies hospitalized for ovarian hyperstimulation syndrome: A case-control study. *Fertility and Sterility*. 2011;95:1629–1632.

8. Halliday J. Outcomes of IVF conceptions: Are they different? *Best Practice & Research. Clinical Obstetrics & Gynaecology*. 2007;21:67–81.

9. Ananth CV, Peedicayil A, Savitz DA. Effect of hypertensive diseases in preg-nancy on birthweight, gestational duration, and small-for-gestational-age births. *Epidemiology*. 1995;6:391–395.

10. Ahmad AS, Samuelsen SO. Hypertensive disorders in pregnancy and fetal death at different gestational lengths: A population study of 2,121,371 pregnancies. *BJOG: An International Journal of Obstetrics and Gynaecology*. 2012;119: 1521–1528.

11. De Lange TE, Budde MP, Heard AR, Tucker G, Kennare R, Dekker GA. Avoidable risk factors in perinatal deaths: A perinatal audit in South Australia. *The Australian & New Zealand Journal of Obstetrics & Gynaecology*. 2008;48:50–57.

12. Hart R, Norman RJ. The longer-term health outcomes for children born as a result of IVF treatment: Part I – general health outcomes. *Human Reproduction Update*. 2013;19:232–243.

13. Helmerhorst FM, Perquin DA, Donker D, Keirse MJ. Perinatal outcome of single-tons and twins after assisted conception: A systematic review of controlled studies. *BMJ*. 2004;328:261.

14. Redman CW, Sargent IL. Latest advances in understanding preeclampsia. *Science*. 2005;308:1592–1594.

15. Healy DL, Breheny S, Halliday J, Jaques A, Rushford D, Garrett C, Talbot JM, Baker HW. Prevalence and risk factors for obstetric haemorrhage in 6730 singleton births after assisted reproductive technology in Victoria Australia. *Human Reproduction*. 2010;25:265–274.

16. Jaques AM, Amor DJ, Baker HW, Healy DL, Ukoumunne OC, Breheny S, Garrett C, Halliday JL. Adverse obstetric and perinatal outcomes in subfertile women conceiv-ing without assisted reproductive technologies. *Fertility and Sterility*. 2010;94: 2674–2679.

17. van der Hoorn ML, Lashley EE, Bianchi DW, Claas FH, Schonkeren CM, Scherjon SA. Clinical and immunologic aspects of egg donation pregnancies: A systematic review. *Human Reproduction Update*. 2010;16:704–712.

18. Jauniaux E, Ben-Ami I, Maymon R. Do assisted-reproduction twin pregnancies require additional antenatal care? *Reproductive Biomedicine Online*. 2013;26:107–119.

19. Bhatt-Mehta V, Deluga KS. Fetal exposure to lisinopril: Neonatal manifestations and management. *Pharmacotherapy.* 1993;13:515–518.

20. Tabacova SA, Kimmel CA. Enalapril: Pharmacokinetic/dynamic inferences for comparative developmental toxicity. A review. *Reproductive Toxicology.* 2001;15:467–478.

21. Magee LA, Abalos E, von Dadelszen P, Sibai B, Easterling T, Walkinshaw S, Group CS. How to manage hypertension in pregnancy effectively. *British Journal of Clinical Pharmacology.* 2011;72:394–401.

22. Magee LA, von Dadelszen P, Chan S, Gafni A, Gruslin A, Helewa M, Hewson S, Kavuma E, Lee SK, Logan AG, McKay D, Moutquin JM, Ohlsson A, Rey E, Ross S, Singer J, Willan AR, Hannah ME, Group CPTC. The control of hypertension in pregnancy study pilot trial. *BJOG: An International Journal of Obstetrics and Gynaecology.* 2007;114:770, e713–e720.

23. Abalos E, Duley L, Steyn DW, Henderson-Smart DJ. Antihypertensive drug therapy for mild to moderate hypertension during pregnancy. *The Cochrane Database of Systematic Reviews.* 2007:CD002252.

24. Abramov Y, Elchalal U, Schenker JG. Obstetric outcome of *in vitro* fertilized pregnancies complicated by severe ovarian hyperstimulation syndrome: A multicenter study. *Fertility and Sterility.* 1998;70:1070–1076.

25. Wiser A, Levron J, Kreizer D, Achiron R, Shrim A, Schiff E, Dor J, Shulman A. Outcome of pregnancies complicated by severe ovarian hyperstimulation syndrome (OHSS): A follow-up beyond the second trimester. *Human Reproduction.* 2005;20:910–914.

26. van Disseldorp J, Eijkemans R, Fauser B, Broekmans F. Hypertensive pregnancy complications in poor and normal responders after *in vitro* fertilization. *Fertility and Sterility.* 2010;93:652–657.

27. Duley L, Henderson-Smart DJ, Knight M, King JF. Antiplatelet agents for preventing pre-eclampsia and its complications. *The Cochrane Database of Systematic Reviews.* 2004:CD004659.

28. Groeneveld E, Lambers MJ, Lambalk CB, Broeze KA, Haapsamo M, de Sutter P, Schoot BC, Schats R, Mol BW, Hompes PG. Preconceptional low-dose aspirin for the prevention of hypertensive pregnancy complications and preterm delivery after IVF: A meta-analysis with individual patient data. *Human Reproduction.* 2013;28:1480–1488.

29. Hofmeyr GJ, Duley L, Atallah A. Dietary calcium supplementation for prevention of pre-eclampsia and related problems: A systematic review and commentary. *BJOG: An International Journal of Obstetrics and Gynaecology.* 2007;114:933–943.

30. Poston L, Briley AL, Seed PT, Kelly FJ, Shennan AH, Vitamins in Pre-eclampsia Trial C. Vitamin C and vitamin E in pregnant women at risk for pre-eclampsia (VIP trial): Randomised placebo-controlled trial. *Lancet.* 2006;367:1145–1154.

31. Bellamy L, Casas JP, Hingorani AD, Williams DJ. Pre-eclampsia and risk of cardiovascular disease and cancer in later life: Systematic review and meta-analysis. *BMJ.* 2007;335:974.

32. Kaaja RJ, Greer IA. Manifestations of chronic disease during pregnancy. *JAMA: The Journal of the American Medical Association.* 2005;294:2751–2757.

33. van Rijn BB, Nijdam ME, Bruinse HW, Roest M, Uiterwaal CS, Grobbee DE, Bots ML, Franx A. Cardiovascular disease risk factors in women with a history of early-onset preeclampsia. *Obstetrics and Gynecology.* 2013;121:1040–1048.

34. Veltman-Verhulst SM, van Rijn BB, Westerveld HE, Franx A, Bruinse HW, Fauser BC, Goverde AJ. Polycystic ovary syndrome and early-onset preeclampsia: Reproductive manifestations of increased cardiovascular risk. *Menopause.* 2010;17:990–996.
35. Barker DJ. Adult consequences of fetal growth restriction. *Clinical Obstetrics and Gynecology.* 2006;49:270–283.

8

The Patient with Obesity

T Hardy and W Ledger

CONTENTS

KEY WORDS: *obesity, metabolic syndrome, polycystic ovary syndrome, BMI, Barker hypothesis, weight loss*

Introduction

Obesity has emerged as one of the central public health concerns of the twenty-first century. Apart from the well-documented effects on metabolic health in adulthood, excess body weight has a range of negative effects on reproductive outcomes, including perinatal and intergenerational effects on offspring health. Importantly, such effects can be mediated through not only the female but also the male partner, giving further impetus to strategies aimed at improving the metabolic health of the couple as a unit. This chapter reviews the effects of this increasingly common problem on outcomes in natural and assisted reproduction and offers an approach to the management of the obese patient in the IVF clinic.

Background

Excess body weight has been defined by the World Health Organisation (WHO)[1] using the body mass index (BMI) categories of overweight (>25.0 kg/m²), obese (>30.0 kg/m²) and severe (>35 kg/m²) and morbid obesity (>40 kg/m²), although these values have been validated in the Caucasian population and lower values may be necessary to account for racial and ethnic differences.[2] Other measures of body weight and composition can be used to more accurately define the distribution of excess body fat, the most commonly used being the waist-to-hip ratio (WHR) which has a stronger correlation with metabolic risk and long-term disease.[3] Together, these measures can provide a rapid categorisation of the individual into metabolic risk categories and allow intra-individual and inter-individual comparisons for clinical and research purposes.

Officially defined in 1997 as a worldwide epidemic,[1] the levels of obesity worldwide have increased in association with dietary, behavioural and socioeconomic changes which have combined increases in the energy composition of food with the uptake of a sedentary lifestyle.[4] Current figures suggest that 1.1–1.7 billion adults and 10% of children worldwide are overweight or obese.[2] In the reproductive age population, greater than 50% of women in the United Kingdom[3] and Australia[5] and greater than 60% in the United States[6] are overweight or obese. There are significant direct and indirect costs to the health system and economy associated with obesity and associated metabolic complications, with the direct health costs projected to reach 16–18% of total health care expenditure by 2030 in the United States.[6]

It is well recognised that excess body weight (BMI > 25) is associated with an increased risk of a range of metabolic and vascular complications, certain cancers, and other nonfatal but disabling conditions (Table 8.1). In particular, there is a strong association between excess body weight and the metabolic syndrome, which may present in younger women in association with polycystic ovary syndrome[7] (PCOS) and in older patients with increased all-cause mortality.[8] Women with PCOS may have an increased propensity to develop obesity, and appropriate investigation should be undertaken to rule out PCOS in the obese patient given the different focus to management.[9]

TABLE 8.1

Comorbidities Associated with BMI > 25.0 kg/m²

Metabolic and Vascular Complications	Cancer	Other
Essential hypertension	Breast	Infertility
Hypercholesterolaemia	Colon	Pregnancy complications
Diabetes	Endometrial	Impairment of offspring metabolic health
Obstructive sleep apnoea	Kidney	Osteoarthritis
Coronary artery disease	Oesophageal	Asthma
Cerebrovascular disease	Gallbladder	

Impact of Disease on IVF and Pregnancy

Female Obesity

Body weight and composition play a central role in determining readiness for the pubertal transition and adult reproductive function.[10] The association between body weight and early maturation was first demonstrated in the mid-twentieth century,[11] and it has since become clear that extremes of body weight are negatively associated with reproductive function, with higher rates of infertility, miscarriage, recurrent miscarriage and pregnancy complications in overweight and obese patients.[12] However, although female overweight and obesity do have a negative impact on a variety of reproductive parameters, it is worth noting that the majority of obese women remain fertile,[13] perhaps due to an evolutionary bias against the underweight end of the body weight spectrum.

Female obesity leads to a reduction in fecundity in both anovulatory and ovulatory patients,[14] with an increased time to pregnancy (>12 months) in natural cycles (odds ratio [OR] 1.32 for women and OR 1.19 for men).[15] Obesity is a known risk factor for anovulatory dysfunction, which commonly manifests as part of PCOS.[3] Although not all women with PCOS are overweight or obese, the conditions share common pathways in their effect on reproductive function through alterations in reproductive hormone profiles and insulin resistance.[10] In addition, overweight and obese women with normal ovulatory cycles also have increased rates of subfertility.[16] This may be due to endometrial changes causing a higher risk of miscarriage, with the oocyte donation model demonstrating miscarriage rates in obese recipients significantly higher than counterparts with normal weight (38.1% vs. 13.3%).[17] In a later study analysing 9,587 oocyte donation cycles over a 12-year period, the same group reported significantly reduced implantation, clinical pregnancy and live birth rates between lean/normoweight and overweight/obese patients,[18] confirming their earlier suggestion that IVF outcomes are not impaired due to effects on embryo quality.[19] This is further supported by the finding that patients with obesity are more likely to have euploid first trimester miscarriages than the normal weight population.[20]

In women undergoing assisted reproductive treatment, excess body weight has also been associated with increased cycle cancellation rates, decreased clinical pregnancy rates and lower live birth rates when compared with women of normal weight.[21,22] Miscarriage rates were also higher in overweight patients undergoing IVF (38% vs. 20%).[23] Increasing obesity was associated with a significant difference in clinical pregnancy in autologous oocyte cycles, suggesting a possible effect of the adverse hormonal and metabolic environment on oocyte quality and embryo development.[24] Overall, patients with a BMI > 30 have up to 68% lower odds of live birth following assisted reproductive treatment compared with women with BMI < 30,[25] although effects are seen in the overweight (BMI > 25) population as well.[26]

Male Obesity

Although the effects of excess body fat in the female have been well studied, attention has only recently shifted to the effects of male obesity on reproductive and offspring outcomes.[13] Overweight and obese men have an altered reproductive hormone profile, with a reduction in serum testosterone levels and increased oestrogen production by aromatization of androgens in peripheral fat.[27,28] The effect on semen quality as measured by conventional parameters is controversial, with some authors suggesting an increased incidence of oligozoospermia and asthenozoospermia in overweight and obese men,[29–33] while others argue the differences are marginal at best.[34,35] In the assisted reproductive setting, increased paternal BMI has no apparent effect on early embryo development[36,37] but has been shown to reduce development to the blastocyst stage and subsequent clinical pregnancy rates and live birth rates.[38]

Pregnancy and Offspring Outcomes

Apart from a higher miscarriage rate regardless of the mode of conception,[39] adverse intrapartum and perinatal outcomes are more common in the overweight and obese population.[40] Overweight and obese women have an increased risk of pre-eclampsia, gestational diabetes, macrosomia, gestational hypertension, thromboembolic disorders, shoulder dystocia, meconium aspiration, intrauterine fetal death, neonatal death, fetal distress and caesarean delivery.[41,42] The risk of preterm birth is also significantly raised in the obese population.[43] Additionally, the risk of congenital malformations (including ventral wall defects, neural tube defects, cardiac defects and multiple congenital anomalies) is significantly increased in the obese population.[44] Proposed explanations for these findings include hyperglycemia, hyperinsulinemia or coexisting diabetes mellitus, and dietary vitamin deficiencies, all of which are associated with birth defects. Perhaps of greater relevance to the developing obesity epidemic, there may be an impact of maternal obesity on childhood and adult health through developmental programming in utero, as suggested in the Barker hypothesis.[45] These effects may also be mediated through the male partner, with recent animal studies demonstrating alterations in microRNA profiles that were associated with changes in the metabolic health of offspring.[46] These findings underlie the importance of improving the health of both partners in order to ameliorate the effect on offspring health, especially given that many couples may not realise there is such an effect.[47]

Impact of IVF and Pregnancy on Disease

IVF is not a risk factor for obesity per se, although the significant psychological stress of undergoing assisted reproductive treatment may exacerbate the lifestyle structures contributing to weight gain in overweight and obese patients or may contribute negatively to the psychological health of the overweight or obese woman. Pregnancy itself is a risk factor for the development of obesity, with many women becoming overweight or obese during pregnancy and not returning to their pre-pregnancy weight postnatally.[48] Women should be aware of the fact that a small increase in BMI between pregnancies can be responsible for a significant increase in the risk of obstetric complications in subsequent pregnancies.[5]

Preparing the Patient for IVF

Medical practitioners involved in the care of reproductive age women should emphasise the importance of lifestyle change and weight loss in all women who are overweight or obese, as the majority will not present to IVF clinics despite their increased need for reproductive assistance. The IVF setting provides a unique opportunity to offer preconception counselling and initiate lifestyle changes in the couple that can significantly improve their reproductive prospects and obstetric outcomes.[49] Attention to the possible comorbidities of obesity prior to initiation of assisted reproductive treatment, especially those with a possible effect on reproductive outcomes and off-spring health (e.g. type II diabetes mellitus), will allow early referral to appropriate medical services and ensure an optimal environment for conception.

The key questions in management prior to initiating an IVF cycle are:

1. Which dietary and lifestyle changes have the most evidence for improving outcomes in overweight and obese patients?
2. Which medical and surgical therapies are safe and effective in the preconception period?
3. Should there be limits to the provision of IVF services in the overweight or obese patient?

Dietary and lifestyle modification remains the cornerstone for treatment of excess body weight. Women should be informed that reducing their BMI will increase their chances of conceiving naturally and with assisted reproduction and be encouraged to participate in a group program as this is more effective than weight loss counselling alone.[50] Dietary advice should centre on reducing caloric intake, with the most important factor determining success being consistent adherence to the dietary plan rather than the particulars of the plan.[51] Patients should aim for at least a 5–10% weight loss and ideally a return to normal BMI range, with the assistance of a dietitian if necessary.[52] The importance of dietary quality should be stressed with adequate intake of protein, fruit and vegetables and avoidance of high-energy foods.[2] Very low calorie diets have high rates of dropout and should not be recommended.[53] Exercise advice should be individually tailored but generally includes daily exercise of moderate intensity and an encouragement of incidental exercise.[5] Weight loss is particularly effective in anovulatory patients but should be encouraged in all patients as reproductive outcomes improve regardless of the cause of subfertility.[54–56] However, there is disagreement over the value of short-term weight loss in improving clinical outcomes,[57,58] and patients should be supported in achieving sustained weight loss.[59]

Pharmacotherapy can be considered in the management of the significantly obese patient but is not a replacement for appropriate dietary and lifestyle modification. A meta-analysis of available medical therapies for weight loss found a modest increase (up to 4.0 kg) in weight loss compared with placebo alone.[60] Tested agents include appetite suppressants such as sibutramine[61] and phentermine,[13] insulin-sensitising agents such as metformin,[62] anti-absorptive agents such as orlistat,[62] and cannabinoid receptor antagonists such as rimonabant (which was withdrawn due to adverse side effects).[63] When using these medications, consideration must be given to local guidelines, patient acceptability, cost and possible teratogenic outcomes given the overall lack of data in the reproductive population (sibutramine and phentermine, for example, are pregnancy category C and therefore not recommended).[13]

Experience with bariatric surgery has been positive in terms of achieving weight loss and reversing metabolic complications in obese patients, and early data from the reproductive population suggest an improvement in fertility rates and pregnancy outcomes.[64,65] It is generally considered for patients with a BMI > 40.0 kg/m^2 and includes bypass (Roux-en-Y) or banding approaches, of which bypass is more effective in achieving weight loss but carries higher perioperative risks.[66] Given the increasing utilisation of bariatric surgery, it is important that clinicians are aware of the indications for referral to bariatric surgical services.[67] Women should be discouraged from trying to conceive during the rapid weight loss phase after bariatric surgery as the attendant metabolic changes may not be conducive to healthy pregnancy.

There has been some consideration of limiting the provision of IVF services to women above a certain BMI cutoff, given the association with poor IVF outcomes and the attendant pregnancy complications when conception is achieved.[68] However, it is more appropriate for clinicians involved in providing IVF to overweight and obese patients to take responsibility for optimising their preconception health through a structured program and referral to appropriate medical and surgical colleagues, as necessary.[49]

Management during IVF Treatment

The pertinent issues surrounding IVF treatment in the overweight or obese patient include increased gonadotrophin requirements, higher cycle cancellation rates, lower peak estradiol levels, oocyte number and maturation.[69–73] Obese patients may have a decreased response to controlled ovarian stimulation despite requiring much higher overall gonadotrophin doses and longer periods of ovarian stimulation.[74] No difference has been demonstrated between antagonist and long agonist protocols in obese patients.[75] The ovarian stimulation protocol, gonadotrophin starting level and further dosage should therefore be individualised in accordance with BMI and other relevant factors and close monitoring of follicle development and estradiol levels undertaken as per standard protocol.[50]

Consideration should be given to the difficulties in performing procedures such as oocyte retrieval and embryo transfer in obese patients, with appropriate facilities (including ultrasound guidance of embryo transfer) and experienced staff often required to achieve satisfactory outcomes.[71] Most clinicians report transferring the same number of embryos regardless of BMI, an appropriate strategy given the increased risks associated with multiple pregnancy in the overweight and obese population.[52] Arguably, single embryo transfer should be considered mandatory in this population to limit the obstetric complications of multiple pregnancy. Patients can be reassured that there is no data to suggest an association between excess body weight and common complications of assisted reproductive techniques (ARTs) such as ectopic and multiple pregnancy and ovarian hyperstimulation syndrome (OHSS; although the diagnosis of PCOS should have been excluded as part of the workup, as this will alter the risk of OHSS).[76]

Management in Early Pregnancy

In obese patients who have conceived naturally, a dating ultrasound early in the first trimester is appropriate given the prevalence of menstrual irregularity in this group and the increased risk of multiple pregnancy.[77] Further ultrasound examinations may need to be undertaken in a specialist centre given the increased risk of fetal anomalies, difficulty clinically detecting intrauterine growth retardation and the challenges of scanning due to maternal body habitus.[5] Advice regarding appropriate weight gain in pregnancy according to WHO criteria should be given early in pregnancy (Table 8.2)[5] and patients encouraged to continue with the dietary and lifestyle changes achieved in the

TABLE 8.2

Recommended Weight Gain in Singleton Pregnancy

BMI Range (kg/m²)	Recommended Weight Gain (kg)
Normal (19.0–24.9)	11.0–16.0
Overweight (25.0–29.9)	7.0–11.0
Obese class 1 (30.0–34.9)	4.0–11.0
Obese class 2 (35.0–39.9)	0.0–4.0
Obese class 3 (>40.0)	0.0-kg weight gain or up to 4.0-kg weight loss

preconception period.[77] Referral to an antenatal care service with appropriate obstetric, medical and surgical facilities may be necessary depending on the degree of obesity.[5]

Conclusion

Obesity is a significant public health issue with ramifications in terms of reproductive and obstetric outcomes and offspring health. Clinicians should take responsibility in ensuring that patients accessing IVF services are appropriately counselled about the risks of excess body weight and strategies to reduce their weight. Patients should be given all necessary support to achieve weight loss prior to IVF, as the increased motivation to achieve health gains in the pre-pregnancy period presents a significant opportunity to improve their reproductive and long-term health.

Key Management Points

1. Presentation for assisted reproduction offers an excellent opportunity for clinicians to improve the preconception health and maximise obstetric outcomes in the obese patient.
2. Patients should undergo a preconception health assessment, including a measurement of BMI and WHR, as well as consideration of alternative diagnoses such as PCOS.
3. Both male and female obesity have a negative impact on reproductive outcomes, and the couple should be treated as a unit.
4. Dietary and lifestyle modification remains the cornerstone for treatment of excess body weight. Consistent adherence to a dietary plan is more important than the particulars of the plan itself.
5. Medical and surgical approaches to the management of obesity are increasingly utilised, especially bariatric surgery. Referral to specialist practitioners should be considered in appropriate patients.
6. Obese patients require higher gonadotrophin doses and consideration must be given to the increased difficulty in performing procedures such as oocyte retrieval and embryo transfer.
7. Single embryo transfer is the gold standard practice for the limitation of complications of multiple pregnancy and should be strongly advised in the obese patient.

8. Patients should be advised regarding early dating ultrasound, appropriate weight gain in pregnancy and specialist obstetric care due to the increased rate of pregnancy complications in obese patients.

REFERENCES

1. World Health Organisation. *Obesity: Preventing and managing the global epidemic.* WHO Technical Report Series Number 894. Geneva: WHO, 2000.
2. Haslam DW, James WP. Obesity. *Lancet.* 2005;366:1197–209.
3. Balen AH, Anderson RA, Policy and Practice Committee of the BFS. Impact of obesity on female reproductive health: British Fertility Society, policy and practice guidelines. *Hum Fertil (Camb).* 2007;10:195–206.
4. Lawlor DA, Bedford C, Taylor M, et al. Geographical variation in cardiovascular disease, risk factors, and their control in older women: British Women's Heart and Health Study. *J Epidemiol Community Health.* 2003;57:134–140.
5. Royal Australian and New Zealand College of Obstetricians and Gynaecologists. *Management of obesity in pregnancy.* College Statement C-Obs 49, March 2013. Melbourne: Royal Australian and New Zealand College of Obstetricians and Gynaecologists.
6. Wang YC, McPherson K, Marsh T, et al. Health and economic burden of the projected obesity trends in the USA and the UK. *Lancet.* 2011;378:815–25.
7. Moran LJ, Misso ML, Wild RA, et al. Impaired glucose tolerance, type 2 diabetes and metabolic syndrome in polycystic ovary syndrome: A systematic review and meta-analysis. *Hum Reprod Update.* 2010;16:347–63.
8. Trevisan M, Liu J, Bahsas FB, et al. Syndrome X and mortality: A population-based study. Risk Factor and Life Expectancy Research Group. *Am J Epidemiol.* 1998; 148:958–66.
9. Glueck CJ, Dharashivkar S, Wang P, et al. Obesity and extreme obesity, manifest by ages 20–24 years, continuing through 32–41 years in women, should alert physicians to the diagnostic likelihood of polycystic ovary syndrome as a reversible underlying endocrinopathy. *Eur J Obstet Gynecol Reprod Biol.* 2005;122:206–12.
10. Bohler H, Mokshagundam S, Winters SJ. Adipose tissue and reproduction in women. *Fertil Steril.* 2010;94:795–825.
11. Davies MJ. Evidence for effects of weight on reproduction in women. *Reprod Biomed Online.* 2006;12:552–61.
12. Bellver J. Obesity and poor reproductive outcome: Female and male body weight matter. *Fertil Steril.* 2013;99:1558–9.
13. Practice Committee of American Society for Reproductive Medicine. Obesity and reproduction: An educational bulletin. *Fertil Steril.* 2008;90:S21–9.
14. Gesink Law DC, Maclehose RF, Longnecker MP. Obesity and time to pregnancy. *Hum Reprod.* 2007;22:414–20.
15. Ramlau-Hansen CH, Thulstrup AM, Nohr EA, et al. Subfecundity in overweight and obese couples. *Hum Reprod.* 2007;22:1634–7.
16. van der Steg JW, Steures P, Eijkemans MJ, et al. Obesity affects spontaneous pregnancy chances in subfertile, ovulatory women. *Hum Reprod.* 2008;23:324–8.
17. Bellver J, Rossal LP, Bosch E, et al. Obesity and the risk of spontaneous abortion after oocyte donation. *Fertil Steril.* 2003;79:1136–40.
18. Belver J, Pellicer A, Garcia-Velasco JA, et al. Obesity reduces uterine receptivity: Clinical experience from 9,587 first cycles of ovum donation with normal weight donors. *Fertil Steril.* 2013;100:1050–8.

19. Bellver J, Ayllon Y, Ferrando M, et al. Female obesity impairs *in vitro* fertilization outcome without affecting embryo quality. *Fertil Steril.* 2010;93:447–54.
20. Landres IV, Milki AA, Lathi RB. Karyotype of miscarriages in relation to maternal weight. *Hum Reprod.* 2010;25:1123–6.
21. Luke B, Brown MB, Missmer SA, et al. The effect of increasing obesity on the response to and outcome of assisted reproductive technology: A national study. *Fertil Steril.* 2011;96:820–5.
22. Petersen GL, Schmidt L, Pinborg A, et al. The influence of female and male body mass index on live births after assisted reproductive technology treatment: A nationwide register-based cohort study. *Fertil Steril.* 2013;99:1654–62.
23. Rittenberg V, Sobaleva S, Ahmad A, et al. Influence of BMI on risk of miscarriage after single blastocyst transfer. *Hum Reprod.* 2011;26:2642–50.
24. Luke B, Brown MB, Stern JE, et al. Female obesity adversely affects assisted reproductive technology (ART) pregnancy and live birth rates. *Hum Reprod.* 2011;26:245–52.
25. Moragianni VA, Jones SM, Ryley DA. The effect of body mass index on the outcomes of first assisted reproductive technology cycles. *Fertil Steril.* 2012;98:102–8.
26. Rittenberg V, Seshadri S, Sunkara SK, et al. Effect of body mass index on IVF treatment outcome: An updated systematic review and meta-analysis. *Reprod Biomed Online.* 2011;23:421–39.
27. Aggerholm AS, Thulstrup AM, Toft G, et al. Is overweight a risk factor for reduced semen quality and altered serum sex hormone profile? *Fertil Steril.* 2008;90:619–26.
28. Pauli EM, Legro RS, Demers LM, et al. Diminished paternity and gonadal function with increasing obesity in men. *Fertil Steril.* 2008;90:346–51.
29. Jensen TK, Andersson AM, Jorgensen N, et al. Body mass index in relation to semen quality and reproductive hormones among 1,558 Danish men. *Fertil Steril.* 2004; 82:863–70.
30. Hammiche F, Laven JS, Twigt JM, et al. Body mass index and central adiposity are associated with sperm quality in men of subfertile couples. *Hum Reprod.* 2012;27:2365–72.
31. Hammoud AO, Wilde N, Gibson M, et al. Male obesity and alteration in sperm parameters. *Fertil Steril.* 2008;90:2222–5.
32. Hofny ER, Ali ME, Abdel-Hafex HZ, et al. Semen parameters and hormonal profile in obese fertile and infertile males. *Fertil Steril.* 2010;94:581–4.
33. Stewart TM, Liu DY, Garrett C, et al. Associations between andrological measures, hormones and semen quality in fertile Australian men: Inverse relationship between obesity and sperm output. *Hum Reprod.* 2009;24:1561–8.
34. Chavarro JE, Toth TL, Wright DL, et al. Body mass index in relation to semen quality, sperm DNA integrity, and serum reproductive hormone levels among men attending an infertility clinic. *Fertil Steril.* 2010;93:2222–31.
35. Duits FH, van Wely M, van der Veen F, et al. Healthy overweight male partners of subfertile couples should not worry about their semen quality. *Fertil Steril.* 2010;94:1356–9.
36. Bellver J, Mifsud A, Grau N, et al. Similar morphokinetic patterns in embryos derived from obese and normoweight infertile women: A time-lapse study. *Hum Reprod.* 2013;28:794–800.
37. Colaci DS, Afeiche M, Gaskins AJ, et al. Men's body mass index in relation to embryo quality and clinical outcomes in couples undergoing *in vitro* fertilization. *Fertil Steril.* 2012;98:1193–9.
38. Bakos HW, Henshaw RC, Mitchell M, et al. Paternal body mass index is associated with decreased blastocyst development and reduced live birth rates following assisted reproductive technology. *Fertil Steril.* 2011;95:1700–4.

39. Metwally M, Ong KJ, Ledger WL, et al. Does high body mass index increase the risk of miscarriage after spontaneous and assisted conception? A meta-analysis of the evidence. *Fertil Steril.* 2008;90:714–26.

40. ESHRE Task Force on Ethics and Law, Dondorp W, de Wert G, et al. Lifestyle-related factors and access to medically assisted reproduction. *Hum Reprod.* 2010;25:578–83.

41. Tennant PW, Rankin J, Bell R. Maternal body mass index and the risk of fetal and infant death: a cohort study from the north of England. *Hum Reprod.* 2011;26:1501–11.

42. Cedergren MI. Maternal morbid obesity and the risk of adverse pregnancy outcome. *Obstet Gynecol.* 2004;103:219–24.

43. Dickey RP, Xiong X, Gee RE, et al. Effect of maternal height and weight on risk of preterm birth in singleton and twin births resulting from *in vitro* fertilization: A retrospective cohort study using the Society for Assisted Reproductive Technology Clinic Outcome Reporting System. *Fertil Steril.* 2012;97:349–54.

44. Watkins ML, Rasmussen SA, Honein MA, et al. Maternal obesity and risk for birth defects. *Pediatrics.* 2003;111:1152–8.

45. Barker DJ. The developmental origins of well-being. *Philos Trans R Soc Lond B Biol Sci.* 2004;359:1359–66.

46. Fullston T, Ohlsson Teague EM, Palmer NO, et al. Paternal obesity initiates metabolic disturbances in two generations of mice with incomplete penetrance to the F2 generation and alters the transcriptional profile of testis and sperm microRNA content. *FASEB J.* 2013;27:4226–43.

47. Hammarberg K, Setter T, Norman RJ, et al. Knowledge about factors that influence fertility among Australians of reproductive age: A population-based survey. *Fertil Steril.* 2013;99:502–7.

48. Pasquali R, Pelusi C, Genghini S, et al. Obesity and reproductive disorders in women. *Hum Reprod Update.* 2003;9:359–72.

49. Nelson SM, Fleming RF. The preconceptual contraception paradigm: Obesity and infertility. *Hum Reprod.* 2007;22:912–5.

50. National Institute for Health and Clinical Excellence. *NICE Clinical Guideline 156: Fertility: assessment and treatment for people with fertility problems.* 2013. Available online http://guidance.nice.org.uk/cg156.

51. Dansinger ML, Gleason JA, Griffith JL, et al. Comparison of the Atkins, Ornish, Weight Watchers, and Zone diets for weight loss and heart disease risk reduction: A randomized trial. *JAMA.* 2005;293:43–53.

52. Harris ID, Python J, Roth L, et al. Physicians' perspectives and practices regarding the fertility management of obese patients. *Fertil Steril.* 2011;96:991–2.

53. Tsagareli V, Noakes M, Norman RJ. Effect of a very-low-calorie diet on *in vitro* fertilization outcomes. *Fertil Steril.* 2006;86:227–9.

54. Clark AM, Ledger W, Galletly C, et al. Weight loss results in significant improvement in pregnancy and ovulation rates in anovulatory obese women. *Hum Reprod.* 1995;10:2705–12.

55. Clark AM, Thornley B, Tomlinson L, et al. Weight loss in obese infertile women results in improvement in reproductive outcome for all forms of fertility treatment. *Hum Reprod.*1998;13:1502–5.

56. Norman RJ, Noakes M, Wu R, et al. Improving reproductive performance in overweight/obese women with effective weight management. *Hum Reprod Update.* 2004;10:267–80.

57. Chavarro JE, Ehrlich S, Colaci DS, et al. Body mass index and short-term weight change in relation to treatment outcomes in women undergoing assisted reproduction. *Fertil Steril.* 2012;98:109–16.

58. Moran L, Tsagareli V, Norman R, et al. Diet and IVF pilot study: Short-term weight loss improves pregnancy rates in overweight/obese women undertaking IVF. *Aust N Z J Obstet Gynaecol.* 2011;51:455–9.

59. Pelletier L, Baillargeon JP. Clinically significant and sustained weight loss is achievable in obese women with polycystic ovary syndrome followed in a regular medical practice. *Fertil Steril.* 2010;94:2665–9.

60. Haddock CK, Poston WS, Dill PL, et al. Pharmacotherapy for obesity: A quantitative analysis of four decades of published randomized clinical trials. *Int J Obes Relat Metab Disord.* 2002;26:262–73.

61. Lindholm A, Bixo M, Bjorn I, et al. Effect of sibutramine on weight reduction in women with polycystic ovary syndrome: A randomized, double-blind, placebo-controlled trial. *Fertil Steril.* 2008;89:1221–8.

62. Metwally M, Amer S, Li TC, et al. An RCT of metformin versus orlistat for the management of obese anovulatory women. *Hum Reprod.* 2009;24:966–75.

63. Moran LJ, Pasquali R, Teede HJ, et al. Treatment of obesity in polycystic ovary syndrome: A position statement of the Androgen Excess and Polycystic Ovary Syndrome Society. *Fertil Steril.* 2009;92:1966–82.

64. Sheiner E, Edri A, Balaban E, et al. Pregnancy outcomes of patients who conceive during or after the first year following bariatric surgery. *Am J Obstet Gynecol.* 2011;204:50.

65. Shah DK, Ginsburg ES. Bariatric surgery and fertility. *Curr Opin Obstet Gynecol.* 2010;22:248–54.

66. Scholtz S, Le Roux C, Balen AH. The role of bariatric surgery in the management of female fertility. *Hum Fertil (Camb).* 2010;13:67–71.

67. Merhi ZO. Impact of bariatric surgery on female reproduction. *Fertil Steril.* 2009;92:1501–8.

68. Vahratian A, Smith YR. Should access to fertility-related services be conditional on body mass index? *Hum Reprod.* 2009;24:1532–7.

69. Dodson WC, Kunselman AR, Legro RS. Association of obesity with treatment outcomes in ovulatory infertile women undergoing superovulation and intrauterine insemination. *Fertil Steril.* 2006;86:642–6.

70. Dokras A, Baredziak L, Blaine J, et al. Obstetric outcomes after *in vitro* fertilization in obese and morbidly obese women. *Obstet Gynecol.* 2006;108:61–9.

71. Tamer Erel C, Senturk LM. The impact of body mass index on assisted reproduction. *Curr Opin Obstet Gynecol.* 2009;21:228–35.

72. Fedorcsak P, Dale PO, Storeng R, et al. Impact of overweight and underweight on assisted reproduction treatment. *Hum Reprod.* 2004;19:2523–8.

73. Souter I, Baltagi LM, Kuleta D, et al. Women, weight, and fertility: The effect of body mass index on the outcome of superovulation/intrauterine insemination cycles. *Fertil Steril.* 2011;95:1042–7.

74. Maheshwari A, Scotland G, Bell J, et al. The direct health services costs of providing assisted reproduction services in overweight or obese women: A retrospective cross-sectional analysis. *Hum Reprod.* 2009;24(3):633–9.

75. Kumbak B, Akbas H, Sahin L, et al. Ovarian stimulation in women with high and low body mass index: GnRH agonist versus GnRH antagonist. *Reprod Biomed Online.* 2010;20:314–9.

76. Koning AM, Mutsaerts MA, Kuchenbecker WK, et al. Complications and outcome of assisted reproduction technologies in overweight and obese women. *Hum Reprod.* 2012;27:457–67.

77. Gunatilake RP, Perlow JH. Obesity and pregnancy: clinical management of the obese gravida. *Am J Obstet Gynecol.* 2011;204:106–19.

9

The Patient with Polycystic Ovary Syndrome

SMC De Sousa and RJ Norman

CONTENTS

KEY WORDS: *polycystic ovary syndrome, insulin resistance, androgen excess, polycystic ovaries, anovulatory infertility, obesity, bariatric surgery, ovulation induction, clomiphene citrate, metformin, laparoscopic ovarian surgery, multiple pregnancy, ovarian hyperstimulation syndrome, cardiometabolic risk*

Background

Polycystic ovary syndrome (PCOS) is one of the most common endocrinopathies among women of reproductive age, making it a common cause, or component, of subfertility.[1] The prevalence ranges from 8.7% to 17.8% depending on the clinical criteria used, with over two-thirds of the affected population unaware of their diagnosis.[2] The first of the multiple diagnostic criteria proposed (Table 9.1) was created by the National Institutes of Health in 1990 requiring a combination of irregular anovulatory periods and either hirsutism or raised serum testosterone.[3] The more inclusive Rotterdam criteria require two of three factors to be fulfilled: oligo- or anovulation, clinical and/or biochemical hyperandrogenism, and polycystic ovaries (PCO) on ultrasonography.[4] Both definitions require the exclusion of differential diagnoses such as hyperprolactinaemia and congenital adrenal hyperplasia. More recently, the Androgen Excess–PCOS Society criteria have renewed focus on the hyperandrogenic profile of the condition, requiring clinical and/or biochemical hyperandrogenism in combination with ovarian dysfunction, defined as oligo- or anovulation and/or polycystic ovaries.[5]

TABLE 9.1

Comparison of Different Diagnostic Criteria for PCOS[3–5]

	NIH Criteria 1990	Rotterdam Criteria 2003	AE-PCOS Society Criteria 2006
Criteria requirements	Both	2 of 3	Both
Hyperandrogenism	Clinical or biochemical hyperandrogenism	Clinical or biochemical hyperandrogenism	Clinical or biochemical hyperandrogenism
Ovulatory dysfunction	Chronic oligo- or anovulation	Chronic oligo- or anovulation	Chronic oligo- or anovulation, or polycystic ovaries
		Polycystic ovaries	

Note: AE-PCOS, Androgen Excess–Polycystic Ovary Syndrome Society; NIH, National Institutes of Health.

TABLE 9.2

International Consensus Definition of Polycystic Ovaries by Ultrasound Criteria

- Either of the following required: 12 or more follicles each measuring 2–9 mm in diameter *or* ovarian volume > 10 cm³
- Scan to be repeated during ovarian quiescence if any follicle > 10 mm in diameter
- A single polycystic ovary is sufficient to meet the diagnosis of polycystic ovaries
- Supportive features include increased stromal volume, increased stromal echogenicity and peripherally located follicles, but not necessary for diagnosis

Source: Balen AH, Laven JSE, Tan S, et al. *Human Reprod Update* 2003;9:505–514.
Note: The number of follicles for diagnosis remains debatable.

The 2012 National Institutes of Health Evidence-Based Methodology Workshop on PCOS sought to rectify the conflict between the European and American classifications of PCOS by formally supporting the Rotterdam criteria as the standard of diagnosis.[6] This workshop also focused on the predictive value of particular phenotypes in PCOS, especially the association of PCO with the risk of ovarian hyperstimulation syndrome (OHSS), and the growing need for a new name for PCOS to reflect the heterogeneity of the disease.

PCO in the absence of PCOS is even more prevalent than PCOS and carries a significant risk of OHSS with an odds ratio (OR) of 6.8 (95% CI [confidence interval] 4.9–9.6) found in a meta-analysis of ten studies of women with PCO undergoing assisted reproduction.[7] The diagnosis of PCO, either in isolation or as a component of PCOS, relies on fulfilment of certain criteria on transvaginal ultrasound (Table 9.2),[8] although some controversy persists regarding the number of follicles that qualifies for PCO. Adolescents may be more appropriately investigated via transabdominal ultrasonography.[1] Anti-Mullerian hormone is an emerging non-invasive alternative in identifying women with PCO as it is secreted by granulosa cells and reflects the antral follicle count.[9]

Unlike PCO, a diagnosis of PCOS carries multifaceted health ramifications in addition to its risk of OHSS. Altered reproductive outcomes are a major concern of young women with PCOS and the focus of this chapter. Other manifestations of the disease vary over a woman's lifetime, ranging from cosmetic, psychological and weight concerns in adolescence to long-term complications in later life including type II diabetes mellitus, dyslipidaemia, hypertension, obstructive sleep apnoea and fatty liver disease.[10] PCOS is associated with an increased prevalence of overweight (RR [relative risk] 1.95, 95% CI 1.52–2.50), obesity (RR 2.77, 95% CI 1.33–4.00) and central obesity (RR 1.73, 95% CI 1.31–2.30) further compounding cardiometabolic risk.[11]

Impact of Polycystic Ovary Syndrome on IVF and Pregnancy

The impact of PCOS on pregnancy outcomes was best illustrated in a large meta-analysis published in 2006 by Boomsma et al. looking at 15 case-control studies including 720 women with PCOS and 4505 controls who had conceived naturally or via assisted reproductive technology.[12] Women with PCOS had increased rates of gestational diabetes mellitus (GDM) (OR 2.94, 95% CI 1.70–5.08) and gestational hypertension (OR 3.67, 95% CI 1.98–6.81) that persisted when only analysing 'higher-validity' studies matched for body mass index (BMI), parity and age (Tables 9.3 and 9.4, respectively). The risk of pre-eclampsia was also greater in the PCOS group, though the studies reporting rates of pre-eclampsia involved PCOS populations of lower parity, higher BMI and more frequent multiple gestation compared to controls, all of which affects the baseline risk of pre-eclampsia. Delivery by caesarean section was more common among women with PCOS; however this was not noted in evaluation of higher-validity studies, suggesting that this might have been influenced by

TABLE 9.3

Odds Ratios for Gestational Diabetes Mellitus Comparing Women with PCOS versus Controls

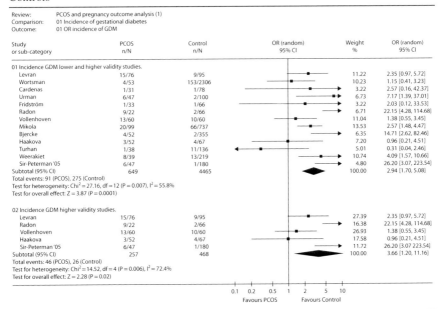

Source: Boomsma CM, Eijkemans MJ, Hughes EG, et al. *Hum Reprod Update* 2006;12:673–683.

TABLE 9.4

Odds Ratios for Gestational Hypertension Comparing Women with PCOS versus Controls

Review: PCOS and pregnancy outcome analysis (1)
Comparison: 04 Incidence of pregnancy induced hypertension
Outcome: 01 OR for incidence PIH

Study or sub-category	PCOS n/N	Control n/N	OR (random) 95% CI	Weight %	OR (random) 95% CI
01 Incidence PIH lower and higher validity studies					
Urman	12/47	8/100		19.33	3.94 [1.49, 10.46]
Fridström	6/33	3/66		11.48	4.67 [1.09, 20.04]
Kashyap	7/22	1/27		5.96	12.13 [1.36, 108.36]
Vollenhoven	10/44	3/44		12.58	4.02 [1.02, 15.79]
Bjercke	6/52	1/355		6.21	46.17 [5.44, 392.13]
Haakova	3/52	4/67		10.55	0.96 [0.21, 4.51]
Turhan	4/38	9/136		14.45	1.66 [0.48, 5.72]
Weerakiet	7/39	15/219		19.42	2.98 [1.13, 7.86]
Subtotal (95% CI)	327	1014		100.00	3.67 [1.98, 6.81]
Total events: 55 (PCOS), 44 (Control)					
Test for heterogeneity: $Chi^2 = 11.30$, df = 7 (P = 0.13), $I^2 = 38.1\%$					
Test for overall effect: Z = 4.13 (P < 0.0001)					
02 Incidence PIH higher validity studies					
Kashyap	7/22	1/27		32.16	12.13 [1.36, 108.36]
Vollenhoven	10/44	3/44		67.84	4.02 [1.02, 15.79]
Subtotal (95% CI)	66	71		100.00	5.48 [1.72, 17.49]
Total events: 17 (PCOS), 4 (Control)					
Test for heterogeneity: $Chi^2 = 0.71$, df = 1 (P = 0.40), $I^2 = 0\%$					
Test for overall effect: Z = 2.87 (P = 0.004)					

0.1   0.2   0.5   1   2   5   10
Favours PCOS   Favours Control

Source: Boomsma CM, Eijkemans MJ, Hughes EG, et al. *Hum Reprod Update* 2006;12:673–683.

maternal obesity. There was a small increase in the rate of premature delivery among women with PCOS, though this was not stratified into spontaneous versus induced delivery, thus the significance of this finding is unclear. Furthermore, while the studies looking at premature delivery reported comparable rates of multiple pregnancy between PCOS subjects and controls, there was significant statistical heterogeneity for this outcome questioning its accuracy.

Neonatal outcomes were also adversely affected by PCOS in the meta-analysis by Boomsma et al. with increased rates of admission to neonatal intensive care and perinatal mortality; however there was no difference in rates of congenital malformations or macrosomia.[12] Because of the small numbers in these outcomes, no comment could be made on differences in BMI, parity or age among these women.

The effects of PCOS on IVF parameters were reviewed in 2006 by Heijnen et al. in a meta-analysis involving 458 women with PCOS and 694 controls spanning nine conventional IVF studies.[13] Women with PCOS had increased cycle cancellation (OR 0.5, 95% CI 0.2–1.0), most likely related to the risks of OHSS and absent or limited ovarian response in the setting of abnormally developed follicles, though the cause was not reported in most studies. While the number of oocytes collected per retrieval was greater among those with PCOS, the total numbers of oocytes fertilised were equivocal. The lower rate of fertilisation in PCOS may be due to an increase of total follicle population with no increase in healthy non-atretic follicles as evidenced by normal inhibin B levels in women with PCOS described elsewhere.[14] PCOS also resulted in longer stimulation periods and a possible increase in severe OHSS. Although there are clear safety concerns when using IVF in PCOS, reproductive success was ultimately comparable to controls with no difference in rates of clinical pregnancy, live birth or miscarriage.[13]

Ovulation induction (OI) and IVF are further complicated in PCOS due to the propensity for multiple gestation. Rates of multiple gestation were reported in only a few of the composite studies of the aforementioned meta-analyses, so the independent effect of PCOS on pregnancy and IVF outcomes is difficult to delineate from the well-established risks of multiple pregnancy.

Impact of IVF and Pregnancy on Polycystic Ovary Syndrome

It is unclear if pregnancy or IVF affects the natural history of PCOS. It is feasible that the weight gain of pregnancy, which persists postpartum in many, may aggravate the long-term health outcomes of women with PCOS. This emphasises the importance of holistic management when seeing women with subfertility due to PCOS.

Preparing the Patient for IVF

Managing subfertility in a woman suspected to have PCOS begins with confirmation of the diagnosis. Clinical assessment involves obtaining a history of oligo- or amenorrhoea and examining for signs of androgen excess. Diagnostic investigations include serum testosterone, sex hormone binding globulin, timed serum progesterone and transvaginal ultrasound. Key differentials should be excluded by testing prolactin, thyroid function, gonadotrophins, basal or adrenocorticotrophic hormone (ACTH)-stimulated 17-OH progesterone for congenital adrenal hyperplasia, 24-hour urinary free cortisol where Cushing's syndrome is suspected and insulin-like growth factor where acromegaly is a differential diagnosis. Attention should be paid to extremely high serum testosterone levels, particularly when associated with elevated DHEA (dehydroepiandrosterone), as this may indicate a virilising neoplasm.[15]

Evaluation for complications should also be conducted at the time of diagnosis of PCOS looking at family history, smoking status, BMI, waist circumference, blood pressure, oral glucose tolerance testing and lipid profile to determine cardiovascular risk as well as pelvic ultrasonography to diagnose endometrial hyperplasia.[16] Women presenting with subfertility should be investigated for additional causes of infertility such as tubal disease or male factors that may favour initial use of IVF.[17]

Women with PCOS who are not actively trying to conceive should be counselled regarding the risk of ovulatory dysfunction. It may be prudent to advise attempting pregnancy at a younger age to improve rates of natural conception and IVF success while reducing the risk of gestational complications seen in women with PCOS. If not seeking fertility, women with PCOS should be advised appropriately regarding contraception especially because of the irregularity of menstrual cycles and the risk of pregnancy in an adverse metabolic environment. In particular, the oral contraceptive pill is attractive because of its restoration of a regular menstrual cycle and beneficial effect on bone health; however small trials suggest that it may exacerbate the insulin resistance that underlies PCOS.[18,19]

Lifestyle Intervention

As the subfertility associated with PCOS is due to ovulatory dysfunction, it is logical that the treatment of choice is restoration of ovulation through lifestyle modification which has been shown to be safe and highly cost effective.[20]

Optimal lifestyle management in PCOS involves a combination of dietary, exercise and behavioural interventions that prevents weight gain and ideally facilitates weight loss. These strategies were demonstrated to improve body composition, clinical and biochemical hyperadrogenism as well as insulin resistance in women with PCOS in a recent Cochrane meta-analysis.[21] Observational studies in obese women with PCOS have additionally illustrated the effectiveness of weight loss in achieving ovulation and possibly also pregnancy.[22,23] As little as 5% weight loss may facilitate pregnancy indicating the feasibility of this treatment strategy,[20,24] although larger weight loss targets are likely required in more marked obesity.

There is insufficient evidence to guide the choice of dietary modification. Studies looking at different diets in PCOS show substantial benefits in hormonal and lipid parameters regardless of dietary composition; however larger randomised controlled trials (RCTs) are needed to elucidate the effects on conception, pregnancy and live birth.[23,25,26] The optimal diet is probably any hypocaloric diet with which the patient can comply.

Exercise-based studies are hampered by a lack of randomisation and employment of counselling services rather than supervised exercise; however an overall increase in physical activity has been shown to reduce the risk of anovulatory infertility in a dose-dependent manner, so this should be advised to all women with PCOS attempting to conceive.[16,27]

Medical and Surgical Weight Loss Strategies

Pharmacotherapy is problematic in obesity due to unacceptable side effects, such as faecal urgency with orlistat and a potential risk of pulmonary hypertension with phentermine.[28] In addition, the safety of these drugs in pregnancy is undetermined. There is increasing evidence of the effectiveness and durability of bariatric surgery in achieving weight loss and treating insulin resistance,[29–31] however there is limited data on reproductive success in the PCOS population. It is nonetheless reasonable to have a low threshold of consideration for such surgery in women of reproductive age with PCOS who are otherwise fit for surgery as this is a disease of obesity and improvements in PCOS parameters have been demonstrated following bariatric surgery.[32] It may be considered if a woman remains at a BMI greater than 35 kg/m^2 after 6 months or longer of lifestyle intervention, provided there is an interim period of at least 12 months during which nutritional deficiencies and other complications of bariatric surgery may be addressed prior to attempting to conceive.[16]

Regardless of the modality used to achieve weight loss, treatment should be enacted prior to attempting to conceive due to concerns of the impact of periconceptional weight loss on pregnancy.[17] Aggressive weight management in the period immediately preceding IVF has been shown to have deleterious effects on reproductive outcomes including cycle cancellation, fertilisation, implantation, ongoing pregnancy and live birth rates.[33] Furthermore, creating an energy deficit periconceptionally may have long-term consequences for the health of offspring as predicted by the 'Barker hypothesis'[34] through various epigenetic changes such as elevated cortisol stress responses identified in more recent animal studies.[35]

Prevention of IVF through Ovulation Induction

In 2007, the American Society for Reproductive Medicine (ASRM) and the European Society for Human Reproduction and Embryology (ESHRE) co-convened a PCOS consensus workshop in Thessaloniki, Greece, the publication of which guides the safe and effective management of OI and IVF in women with PCOS.[17]

The ASRM/ESHRE guidelines recommend clomiphene citrate (CC) as the first-line OI agent.[17] Clinical pregnancy rates were increased by an OR of 5.8 (95% CI 1.6–21.5) in a Cochrane meta-analysis comparing CC to placebo in women with anovulation,[36] the biggest cause of which is PCOS.[1] The ASRM/ESHRE guidelines recommend limiting CC use to 6–12 ovulatory cycles, which has been shown to yield a cumulative conception rate of approximately 60% after six cycles.[37]

The use of metformin for OI either as monotherapy or with CC in women with PCOS was popular for some time prior to a landmark study by Legro et al. in 2007 demonstrating that metformin was inferior to standard OI in women with PCOS, contrary to earlier, smaller studies.[38] This area has since been the subject of multiple Cochrane meta-analyses. The first meta-analysis in 2009 found that metformin did not enhance pregnancy or live birth rates when used before or during IVF/ICSI (intra-cytoplasmic sperm injection) cycles; however it achieved a significant reduction in OHSS (OR 0.27, 95% CI 0.16–0.47).[39] A subsequent Cochrane meta-analysis in 2012 looking at metformin with or without CC found that metformin monotherapy or combination therapy was superior to CC alone in terms of clinical pregnancy rates, but this was found only in the subgroup of women with PCOS who were obese with the greatest benefit seen in women who were CC resistant.[40] There was no difference in live birth rates, questioning the significance of these findings. The ideal duration of metformin-CC combination therapy is also uncertain.[41] The ASRM/ESHRE guidelines currently advise against routine use of this agent in OI, reserving metformin only for women with glucose intolerance.[17]

The standard therapy for OI where women with PCOS are found to be CC resistant is injectable gonadotrophins, typically in a low-dose protocol of 37.5–75 IU of follicle-stimulating hormone (FSH) daily, instead of the usual 150 IU daily, in order to minimise the risk of OHSS.[17] Gonadotrophin stimulation necessitates intensive ultrasound monitoring to document ovulation and predict the risk of multiple pregnancy to facilitate appropriate cycle cancellation.[17] A prospective study looking at 240 women administered CC as first-line therapy and exogenous gonadotrophins as second-line therapy found a cumulative singleton live birth rate of 72%, demonstrating the high success rate of this strategy.[42] Overall, low-dose gonadotrophin regimens result in a mono-ovulation rate of 70%, clinical pregnancy rate of 20% and multiple live birth rate of 6%.[43] The ASRM/ESHRE guidelines recommend that gonadotrophin stimulation be restricted to six cycles.[17]

Laparoscopic ovarian surgery (LOS), by electrocautery or laser vaporisation, is generally considered a third-line therapy for OI.[17] It is typically reserved for CC-resistant cases where the close ultrasound monitoring required for gonadotrophin stimulation is impractical. The mechanism is uncertain, and its evidence is empiric. Success of LOS when used in isolation is modest, with approximately half of women requiring adjuvant CC or exogenous gonadotrophins.[17] However, RCTs comparing LOS to gonadotrophin administration have detected no difference in rates of ongoing pregnancy, miscarriage or live birth, with the advantages of fewer multiple pregnancies and no risk of OHSS in the LOS groups obviating the need for ultrasound monitoring.[44,45]

Management during IVF Treatment

Because of the risk of multiple pregnancy with OI, IVF with single-embryo transfer is considered a viable alternative to improving reproductive success in women with PCOS[17] and might even be preferable to gonadotrophin stimulation in CC-resistant women because of the higher multiple pregnancy rate associated with this agent.[42]

The major concern when employing IVF in PCOS is OHSS. The risk of OHSS may be lessened by utilising low-dose stimulation protocols with a low threshold for cycle cancellation[17] and replacing the human chorionic gonadotrophin (hCG) ovulation trigger with gonadotrophin-releasing hormone (GnRH) agonists. RCTs have shown that GnRH agonist triggers virtually eliminate the risk of OHSS in women with PCO or PCOS.[46,47] A more recent meta-analysis comparing GnRH agonists with the hCG trigger in women with and without PCOS supported this finding of significantly lower rates of OHSS; however this was accompanied by lower birth rates in women given GnRH agonists, suggesting that this technology should be limited to women at high risk of OHSS, such as the PCOS population.[48] Metformin administration during IVF may also reduce the risk of OHSS, as demonstrated by a double-blind RCT looking at 101 IVF/ICSI cycles with OHSS rates of 3.8% in the metformin arm versus 20.4% in the placebo arm ($P = 0.023$).[49] This effect remained significant after adjustment for BMI, age and FSH dose (OR = 0.15, 95% CI 0.03–0.76).

The aforementioned lifestyle measures are also important in the setting of IVF as the goal of weight loss is critical in improving the safety of anaesthesia and reducing pregnancy complications.[12] Even if IVF is required up front, a period of lifestyle modification prior to attempting conception is desirable for these reasons.

Management in Early Pregnancy

Miscarriage rates were traditionally thought to be higher in the setting of PCOS; however these trials tended to have older, more overweight populations.[50,51] No difference in miscarriage rates has been found in more recent PCOS trials.[52–54] In contrast, miscarriage has been shown to be clearly associated with BMI which likely explains the earlier findings.[55]

In addition to its potential role in OI and reducing the risk of OHSS, metformin may improve pregnancy outcomes. In particular, first trimester use of metformin either alone or in combination with OI has been shown to improve clinical pregnancy and live birth rates in a double-blind, placebo-controlled RCT of 320 women, with the most pronounced effect seen in obese women.[54] Metformin was not associated with a change in miscarriage frequency, which is not surprising as miscarriage was not any more common in women with PCOS compared to controls in this study.

Older non-randomised prospective and retrospective studies have suggested that metformin use in PCOS might also reduce the incidence of GDM; however a large double-blind, placebo-controlled RCT by Vanky et al. of 257 women with PCOS disagreed with this, showing no difference in the rates of GDM.[56] There was a benefit of less weight gain in the metformin group, though the value of this in the absence of other clinical differences is uncertain. A subsequent meta-analysis argued that metformin reduced the risk of GDM (OR 0.37, 95% CI 0.25–0.56)[57]; however this result was significantly swayed by prospective cohort studies negating the evidence drawn from the pilot study[58] and final RCT[56] by Vanky et al. which remain the only RCTs in this area to date.

While prospective studies are needed to define precise surveillance protocols, women with PCOS should be considered to have 'at-risk' pregnancies regardless of the method of conception with close monitoring for the established medical complications of GDM, gestational hypertension and possibly pre-eclampsia as well as adverse neonatal outcomes.[12] Postpartum, women should return to regular cardiometabolic risk assessment including annual weight, waist circumference, BMI and blood pressure measurements and two-yearly lipid profile and oral glucose tolerance testing.[16] Early aggressive management of these comorbidities should improve overall health and reproductive outcomes.

Key Management Points

1. Weight loss via lifestyle modification, pharmacotherapy or bariatric surgery may be sufficient to improve fertility in PCOS.

2. OI using clomiphene is effective in preventing the need for IVF, but carries the risk of multiple gestation.

3. Alternative therapies for OI include metformin, exogenous gonadotrophins and LOS.

4. Metformin also improves clinical pregnancy and live birth rates, maternal weight gain and possibly the incidence of GDM.

5. IVF may be required due to failure of OI or other factors of infertility.

6. Ovarian hyperstimulation in women with PCOS undertaking IVF may be avoided via low-dose stimulation protocols, appropriate cycle cancellation, GnRH agonist triggers and metformin.

REFERENCES

1. Norman RJ, Dewailly D, Legro RS, Hickey TE. Polycystic ovary syndrome. *Lancet* 2007;370:685–697.

2. March WA, Moore VM, Willson KJ, et al. The prevalence of polycystic ovary syndrome in a community sample assessed under contrasting diagnostic criteria. *Hum Reprod* 2010;25:544–551.

3. Zawadski JK, Dunaif A. Diagnostic criteria for polycystic ovary syndrome; towards a rational approach. In: Dunaif A, Givens JR, Haseltine R, eds. *Polycystic Ovary Syndrome*. Boston: Blackwell Scientific, 1992:377–384.

4. The Rotterdam ESHRE/ASRM-Sponsored PCOS Consensus Workshop Group. Revised 2003 consensus on diagnostic criteria and long-term health risks related to polycystic ovary syndrome. *Fertil Steril* 2004;81:19–25.

5. Azziz R, Carmina E, Dewailly D, et al. Positions statement: Criteria for defining polycystic ovary syndrome as a predominantly hyperandrogenic syndrome: An Androgen Excess Society guideline. *J Clin Endocrinol Metab* 2006;91:4237–4245.

6. LV DePaolo, chair. Executive summary. In: National Institutes of Health Evidence-Based Methodology Workshop on Polycystic Ovary Syndrome, Bethesda, MD, 2012 December 3–5.

7. Tummon I, Gavrilova-Jordan L, Allemand MC, et al. Polycystic ovaries and ovarian hyperstimulation syndrome: A systematic review. *Acta Obstet Gynecol Scand* 2005;84:611–616.

8. Balen AH, Laven JSE, Tan S, et al. Ultrasound assessment of the polycystic ovary: International consensus definitions. *Human Reprod Update* 2003;9:505–514.

9. Eilertsen TB, Vanky E, Carlsen SM. Anti-Mullerian hormone in the diagnosis of polycystic ovary syndrome: Can morphologic description be replaced? *Hum Reprod* 2012;27:2494–2502.

10. Hardy TS, De Sousa SMC, Norman RJ. Polycystic ovary syndrome: Prognosis and risk of comorbidity. In: Diamanti-Kandarakis E, Nader S, Panidis D, eds. *Novel Insights into the Pathophysiology and Treatment of PCOS*. London: Future Science Group, 2013:2–14.

11. Lim SS, Davies MJ, Norman RJ, et al. Overweight, obesity and central obesity in women with polycystic ovary syndrome: A systematic review and meta-analysis. *Hum Reprod Update* 2012;18:618–637.

12. Boomsma CM, Eijkemans MJ, Hughes EG, et al. A meta-analysis of pregnancy outcomes in women with polycystic ovary syndrome. *Hum Reprod Update* 2006;12:673–683.

13. Heijnen EM, Eijkemans MJ, Hughes EG, et al. A meta-analysis of outcomes of conventional IVF in women with polycystic ovary syndrome. *Hum Reprod Update* 2006;12:13–21.

14. Laven JS, Fauser BC. Inhibins and adult ovarian function. *Mol Cell Endocrinol* 2004;225:37–44.

15. Ehrmann DA. Polycystic ovary syndrome. *N Engl J Med* 2005;352:1223–1236.

16. Jean Hailes Foundation for Women's Health on behalf of the PCOS Australian Alliance. *Evidence-Based Guideline for the Assessment and Management of Polycystic Ovary Syndrome*. Melbourne: National Health and Medical Research Council, 2011.

17. Thessaloniki ESHRE/ASRM PCOS Consensus Workshop Group. Consensus on infertility treatment related to polycystic ovary syndrome. *Human Reprod* 2008;23:462–477.

18. Korytkowski MT, Mokan M, Horwitz MJ, et al. Metabolic effects of oral contraceptives in women with polycystic ovary syndrome. *J Clin Endocrinol Metab* 1995;80:3327–3334.

19. Mastorakos G, Koliopoulos C, Deligeoroglou E, et al. Effects of two forms of combined oral contraceptives on carbohydrate metabolism in adolescents with polycystic ovary syndrome. *Fertil Steril* 2006;85:420–427.

20. Clark AM, Thornley B, Tomlinson L, et al. Weight loss in obese women results in improvement in reproductive outcome for all forms of fertility treatment. *Hum Reprod* 1998;13:1502–1505.

21. Moran LJ, Hutchison SK, Norman RJ, et al. Lifestyle changes in women with polycystic ovary syndrome. *Cochrane Database Syst Rev* 2011;7:CD007506.

22. Clark AM, Ledger W, Galletly C, et al. Weight loss results in significant improvement in pregnancy and ovulation rates in anovulatory obese women. *Hum Reprod* 1995;10:2705–2712.

23. Moran LJ, Pasquali R, Teede HJ, et al. Treatment of obesity in polycystic ovary syndrome: A position statement of the Androgen Excess and Polycystic Ovary Syndrome Society. *Fertil Steril* 2009;92:1966–1982.

24. Kiddy DS, Hamilton-Fairley D, Bush A, et al. Improvement in endocrine and ovarian function during dietary treatment of obese women with polycystic ovary syndrome. *Clin Endocrinol (Oxf)* 1992;36:105–111.

25. Moran LJ, Noakes M, Clifton PM, et al. Dietary composition in restoring reproductive and metabolic physiology in overweight women with polycystic ovary syndrome. *J Clin Endocrinol Metab* 2003;88:812–819.

26. Stamets K, Taylor DS, Kunselman A, et al. A randomized trial of the effects of two types of short-term hypocaloric diets on weight loss in women with polycystic ovary syndrome. *Fertil Steril* 2004;81:630–637.

27. Rich-Edwards JW, Spiegelman D, Garland M, et al. Physical activity, body mass index, and ovulatory disorder infertility. *Epidemiology* 2002;13:184–190.

28. Eckel RH. Nonsurgical management of obesity in adults. *N Engl J Med* 2008;358:1941–1950.

29. Carlsson LMS, Peltonen M, Ahlin S, et al. Bariatric surgery and prevention of type 2 diabetes in Swedish obese subjects. *N Engl J Med* 2012;367:695–704.

30. Mingrone G, Panunzi S, De Gaetano A, et al. Bariatric surgery versus conventional medical therapy for type 2 diabetes. *N Engl J Med* 2012;366:1577–1585.

31. Schauer PR, Kashyap SR, Wolski K, et al. Bariatric surgery versus intensive medical therapy in obese patients with diabetes. *N Engl J Med* 2012;366:1567–1576.

32. Moran LJ, Norman RJ. The effect of bariatric surgery on female reproductive function. *J Clin Endocrinol Metab* 2012;97:4352–4354.

33. Tsagareli V, Noakes M, Norman RJ. Effect of a very-low-calorie diet on *in vitro* fertilization outcomes. *Fertil Steril* 2006;86:227–229.

34. Barker DJ. Fetal programming of coronary heart disease. *Trends Endocrinol Metab* 2002;13:364–368.

35. Zhang S, Rattanatray L, McMillen IC, et al. Periconceptional nutrition and the early programming of a life of obesity or adversity. *Prog Biophys Mol Biol* 2011;106:307–314.

36. Brown J, Farquhar C, Beck J, et al. Clomiphene and anti-oestrogens for ovulation induction in PCOS. *Cochrane Database Syst Rev* 2009;4:CD002249.

37. Kousta E, White DM, Franks S. Modern use of clomiphene citrate in induction of ovulation. *Hum Reprod Update* 1997;3:359–365.

38. Legro RS, Barnhart HX, Schlaff WD, et al. Clomiphene, metformin, or both for infertility in the polycystic ovary syndrome. *N Engl J Med* 2007;356:551–566.

39. Tso LO, Costello MF, Andriolo RB, et al. Metformin treatment before and during IVF or ICSI in women with polycystic ovary syndrome. *Cochrane Database Syst Rev* 2009;2:CD006105.

40. Tang T, Lord JM, Norman RJ, et al. Insulin-sensitising drugs (metformin, rosiglitazone, pioglitazone, D-chiro-inositol) for women with polycystic ovary syndrome, oligo amenorrhoea and subfertility. *Cochrane Database Syst Rev* 2012;5:CD003053.

41. Sinawat S, Buppasiri P, Lumbiganon P, et al. Long versus short course treatment with metformin and clomiphene citrate for ovulation induction in women with PCOS. *Cochrane Database Syst Rev* 2012;10:CD006226.

42. Eijkemans MJ, Imani B, Mulders AG, et al. High singleton live birth rate following classical ovulation induction in normogonadotrophic anovulatory infertility (WHO 2). *Hum Reprod* 2003;18:2357–2362.

43. Homburg R, Howles CM. Low-dose FSH therapy for anovulatory infertility associated with polycystic ovary syndrome: rationale, results, reflections and refinements. *Hum Reprod Update* 1999;5:493–499.

44. Farquhar CM, Williamson K, Gudex G, et al. A randomized controlled trial of laparoscopic ovarian diathermy versus gonadotropin therapy for women with clomiphene citrate-resistant polycystic ovary syndrome. *Fertil Steril* 2002;78:404–411.

45. Bayram N, van Wely M, Kaaijk EM, et al. Using an electrocautery strategy or recombinant follicle stimulating hormone to induce ovulation in polycystic ovary syndrome: randomised controlled trial. *BMJ* 2004;328:192–196.
46. Babayof R, Margalioth EJ, Huleihel M, et al. Serum inhibin A, VEGF and TNF alpha levels after triggering oocyte maturation with GnRH agonist compared with HCG in women with polycystic ovaries undergoing IVF treatment: A prospective randomized trial. *Hum Reprod* 2006;21:1260–1265.
47. Engmann L, DiLuigi A, Schmidt D, et al. The use of gonadotropin-releasing hormone (GnRH) agonist to induce oocyte maturation after cotreatment with GnRH antagonist in high-risk patients undergoing *in vitro* fertilization prevents the risk of ovarian hyperstimulation syndrome: A prospective randomized controlled study. *Fertil Steril* 2008;89:84–91.
48. Youssef MA, Van der Veen F, Al-Inany HG, et al. Gonadotropin-releasing hormone agonist versus hCG for oocyte triggering in antagonist assisted reproductive technology cycles. *Cochrane Database Syst Rev* 2010;11:CD008046.
49. Tang T, Glanville J, Orsi N, et al. The use of metformin for women with PCOS undergoing IVF treatment. *Hum Reprod* 2006;21:1416–1425.
50. Balen AH, Tan SL, MacDougall J, et al. Miscarriage rates following *in vitro* fertilization are increased in women with polycystic ovaries and reduced by pituitary desensitization with buserelin. *Hum Reprod* 1993;8:959–964.
51. Glueck CJ, Wang P, Fontaine RN, et al. Plasminogen activator inhibitor activity: An independent risk factor for the high miscarriage rate during pregnancy in women with polycystic ovary syndrome. *Metabolism* 1999;48:1589–1595.
52. Koivunen R, Pouta A, Franks S, et al. Fecundability and spontaneous abortions in women with self-reported oligo-amenorrhea and/or hirsutism: Northern Finland Birth Cohort 1966 Study. *Hum Reprod* 2008;23:2134–2139.
53. Moll E, Bossuyt PM, Korevaar JC, et al. Effect of clomifene citrate plus metformin and clomifene citrate plus placebo on induction of ovulation in women with newly diagnosed polycystic ovary syndrome: Randomized double blind clinical trial. *BMJ* 2006;332:1485–1489.
54. Morin-Papunen L, Rantala AS, Unkila-Kallio L, et al. Metformin improves pregnancy and live-birth rates in women with polycystic ovary syndrome (PCOS): A multicenter, double-blind, placebo-controlled randomized trial. *J Clin Endocrinol Metab* 2012;97:1492–1500.
55. Wang JX, Davies M, Norman RJ. Body mass and probability of pregnancy during assisted reproduction treatment: Retrospective study. *BMJ* 2000;321:1320–1321.
56. Vanky E, Stridsklev S, Heimstad R, et al. Metformin versus placebo from first trimester to delivery in polycystic ovary syndrome: A randomized, controlled multicenter study. *J Clin Endocrinol Metab* 2010;95:448–455.
57. Zheng J, Shan PF, Gu W. The efficacy of metformin in pregnant women with polycystic ovary syndrome: A meta-analysis of clinical trials. *J Endocrinol Invest* 2013 [Epub ahead of print].
58. Vanky E, Salvesen KA, Heimstad R, et al. Metformin reduces pregnancy complications without affecting androgen levels in pregnant polycystic ovary syndrome women: Results of a randomized study. *Hum Reprod* 2004;19:1734–1740.

10

The Patient with Hydrosalpinx

A Strandell

CONTENTS

Introduction

Tubal factor infertility was the original indication for which *in vitro* fertilization (IVF) was first performed. During the last decades, it has become evident that tubal infertility in general and hydrosalpinx in particular carry a worse prognosis than other infertility factors. The first report from 1994 showed a reduced pregnancy rate and an increased rate of miscarriage in hydrosalpinx patients, as compared to patients with other tubal infertility,[1] and it has been followed by numerous retrospective studies. Initially, the theories focused on the hydrosalpinx fluid, its content and also the possibility of washout of embryos through leakage of fluid through the uterine cavity. A lot of research has been devoted to investigate the hydrosalpinx fluid for possible embryotoxic components and growth-inhibiting factors, but the mechanism through which a hydrosalpinx exerts its negative effects is still obscure.

Several reports have demonstrated inhibitory effects on embryo growth in mice,[2,3] but not in humans,[4] while other studies have shown growth-promoting properties of the hydrosalpinx fluid.[5] Secondary to the hydrosalpinx fluid's influence on the endometrium, the environmental prerequisite for implantation has been studied. The roles of integrins and several cytokines have been elucidated, but the main question as to why embryos do not implant or develop properly has not yet been answered.[6–9] There is certainly a lack of knowledge, and not even the detailed course from the original tubal infection to the fimbrial closing and the exudation of fluid into the tubal lumen is completely understood.

Despite the lack of knowledge on the mechanism, several treatments aimed at removing hydrosalpingeal fluid have been suggested. The effect of salpingectomy has been thoroughly investigated in randomized controlled trials (RCTs), and transvaginal aspiration and laparoscopic tubal occlusion have also been tested in RCTs. Other treatment options such as hysteroscopic tubal occlusion, interventional ultrasound sclerotherapy and salpingostomy have been subjected to study designs of less validity.

Impact of Hydrosalpinx on IVF Outcomes

Several retrospective studies have reported on the adverse IVF outcome in hydrosalpinx patients. The overall effect of hydrosalpinx is a reduction by half in pregnancy rate per fresh embryo transfer, as demonstrated by one meta-analysis of 10 retrospective studies resulting in a common odds ratio (OR) of 0.57 (95% confidence interval [CI] 0.48–0.68).[10] Also, frozen-thawed cycles are impaired in hydrosalpinx patients, with a common OR of 0.39 (95% CI 0.16–0.94) derived from two studies.[1,11] The same meta-analysis showed a doubling in risk for miscarriage in hydrosalpinx patients, common OR 2.3 (95% CI 1.56–3.48), while no increased risk for ectopic pregnancies could be demonstrated.[10] Figure 10.1 summarizes the overall negative impact of hydrosalpinx on IVF outcome.[12–14]

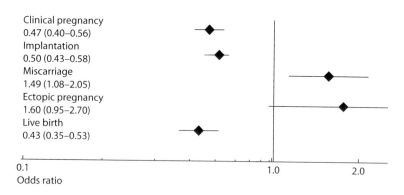

FIGURE 10.1   Meta-analyses of retrospective studies comparing outcomes of IVF in patients with uni- or bilateral hydrosalpinges and controls, showing common odds ratios and 95% confidence intervals, calculated on data from articles included in the latest published meta-analysis and two additional studies. (From Camus E, Poncelet C, Goffinet F, et al. *Hum Reprod* 1999;14:1243–1249; Freeman MR, Whitworth CM, Hill GA. *Hum Reprod* 1998;13:983–986. Murray DL, Sagoskin AW, Widra EA, et al. *Fertil Steril* 1998;69:41–45.)

Impact of Hydrosalpinx Treatment on IVF Outcome

The overwhelming evidence for the negative influence of a hydrosalpinx on IVF outcome started an intense debate about treatment options, most of which focused on surgical methods to dispose of the hydrosalpingeal fluid. Laparoscopic salpingectomy was the first method to be evaluated in RCTs, followed by laparoscopic tubal occlusion and transvaginal aspiration.

Other methods have to be judged taking into account the lower level of evidence.

Salpingectomy

A Scandinavian multicenter study randomized 204 patients to laparoscopic salpingectomy or no intervention prior to the first cycle of IVF.[15] Of special interest were the groups with bilateral and/or ultrasound-visible hydrosalpinges, which were previously shown to have a worse prognosis.[16,17] Patients with ultrasound-visible hydrosalpinges were the ones who benefited most from salpingectomy: live birth rate 40% vs. 17% ($p = 0.04$) without any surgical intervention.[15] The main results from these poor-prognosis groups are shown in Figure 10.2. This study constitutes the major part in a systematic review, including three additional smaller trials on salpingectomy,[18] showing a statistically significant increase in ongoing and clinical pregnancy rates if salpingectomy preceded IVF (OR for ongoing pregnancy rate 2.2, 95% CI 1.3–3.8) in all hydrosalpinx patients. However, the Scandinavian study could demonstrate that the effect was entirely due to the positive effect among those with hydrosalpinges that were enlarged enough to be seen on ultrasound.[19]

The recommendation of salpingectomy has raised concern about unnecessary removal of tubes that might be suitable for salpingostomy and spontaneous conception.

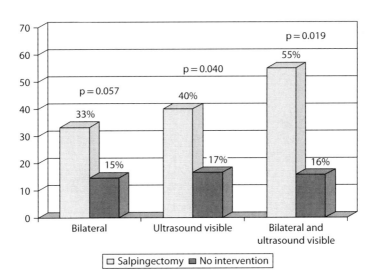

FIGURE 10.2 Live birth rates in the Scandinavian randomized trial of pre-IVF salpingectomy, in groups of patients with bilateral and/or ultrasound-visible hydrosalpinges. (From Strandell A, Lindhard A, Waldenström U, et al. *Hum Reprod* 1999;14:2762–2769.)

The optimal management is of course that the fallopian tube and its mucosal status should be evaluated at the time of laparoscopy, and the immediate decision can be taken whether the tube should be removed or reconstructed. The prerequisite for the latter scenario is surgical/laparoscopic competence for distal tubal repair and also postoperative time to allow for spontaneous conception.

Also, in cases of salpingectomy for unilateral hydrosalpinx, time for spontaneous conception should be considered since several case series have demonstrated the occurrence of spontaneous pregnancies after surgery. A multi-centre study demonstrated that out of 18 women with a mean 2.6 (SD 1.6) years of infertility and a unilateral hydrosalpinx, 16 conceived spontaneously within a mean 3.1 (SD 2.8) months after unilateral salpingectomy.[20]

Tubal Occlusion

Proximal occlusion of the fallopian tube has been suggested as an alternative to salpingectomy, in particular when dense adhesions complicate an intended salpingectomy. Occlusion of the tube serves the purpose of interrupting the passage of fluid to the endometrial cavity but leaves the hydrosalpinx in place, where it might interfere with the aspiration of oocytes.

Laparoscopic Tubal Occlusion

The laparoscopic tubal occlusion procedure can be combined with distal fenestration of the hydrosalpinx, but the opening frequently reoccludes. One underpowered RCT has demonstrated borderline statistical significance for beneficial effect of laparoscopic tubal occlusion (OR for ongoing pregnancy was 7.2 [95% CI 0.9–59.6]).[21] The Cochrane review included one additional RCT, presented only as an abstract.[18] The common OR was then 4.7 (95% CI 2.2–10.0), and it was concluded that laparoscopic tubal occlusion is an alternative to laparoscopic salpingectomy in improving IVF pregnancy rates in women with hydrosalpinges.

The Cochrane review also presented a direct comparison between laparoscopic salpingectomy and laparoscopic tubal occlusion including two small RCTs.[18] The OR for clinical pregnancy rate was 1.28 (95% CI 0.76–2.14) favoring salpingectomy, but the total sample size was too small to conclude that any method was better or equally effective.

Also unilateral tubal occlusion has been reported to increase the possibility of spontaneous conception. In the largest case series, 6/7 conceived in mean within 12.3 (SD 6.7) months.[20]

Hysteroscopic Tubal Occlusion

In cases where salpingectomy or laparoscopy is contraindicated, the hysteroscopic route has been suggested for tubal occlusion. The most commonly reported technique is the placement of the Essure® device, which is an expanding spring device indicated for tubal sterilization. The procedure is typically performed in an ambulatory setting without anaesthesia, but with the use of local analgesia if needed. To date there are less than 100 patients reported in case series, demonstrating feasibility of the technique and pregnancies/live births after subsequent IVF.[22–25] One of the largest series reported successful placement in 19/20 patients and no complications.[23] The cumulative live birth rate per patient was 63%, and the cumulative live birth rate per transfer was 27%. Others have reported a case of reactivated infection, requiring bilateral adnexectomy six months after the procedure.[25] One spontaneous pregnancy after unilateral placement was reported.[25]

There is a need for comparative data to prove the method's efficacy and safety. At the time of writing, an RCT comparing Essure® placement to salpingectomy is ongoing.

One RCT has compared the feasibility of another hysteroscopic technique, using roller ball coagulation, with laparoscopic tubal occlusion.[26] Hysteroscopic access and tubal occlusion was achieved in 9/14 cases. No information on outcomes from subsequent IVF was available.

Transvaginal Aspiration

Ultrasound-guided transvaginal aspiration has been advocated as a treatment option to remove the hydrosalpingeal fluid. If the procedure is performed prior to stimulation, the fluid always reaccumulates. Even if it is done at the time of oocyte retrieval, the risk of recurrence is already high at the time of transfer. Two RCTs have compared transvaginal aspiration of hydrosalpingeal fluid after oocyte retrieval with no aspiration.[27,28] One of them was stopped in advance ($n = 66$) and failed to show benefit,[27] while the other ($n = 110$) demonstrated increased implantation (18.7% vs. 8.3%, $p = 0.023$), clinical pregnancy (31.5% vs. 13.2%, $p = 0.023$) and ongoing pregnancy rate (27.8% vs. 9.4%, $p = 0.015$) after aspiration compared with no aspiration.[28] A negative impact from recurrence of hydrosalpingeal fluid as well as from the appearance of endometrial fluid was also suggested. A meta-analysis of the two published studies on aspiration versus no aspiration of hydosalpingeal fluid demonstrates beneficial effect of aspiration on clinical pregnancy rate (OR 2.6, 95% CI 1.2–5.5), (Figure 10.3).

Transvaginal aspiration has the advantage of being less invasive than a laparoscopic salpingectomy or tubal occlusion. There are however no studies that have made direct comparisons between transvaginal aspiration and laparoscopic methods. There is also a concern about the risk of infection subsequent to a puncture of a hydrosalpinx, and antibiotic coverage is routine. However, infections seem to be very rare, and in the two RCTs, only one positive culture and no infection were reported from a total of 176 patients.[27,28]

Study or Subgroup	Aspiration Events	Aspiration Total	No aspiration Events	No aspiration Total	Weight	Odds Ratio M-H, Fixed, 95% CI	Year
Hammadieh 2008	10	32	6	34	45.2%	2.12 [0.67, 6.74]	2008
Fouda & Sayed 2011	17	54	7	53	54.8%	3.02 [1.13, 8.05]	2011
Total (95% CI)		86		87	100.0%	2.61 [1.24, 5.51]	
Total events	27		13				

Heterogeneity: Chi² = 0.21, df = 1 (P = 0.65); I² = 0%
Test for overall effect: Z = 2.52 (P = 0.01)

Odds Ratio M-H, Fixed, 95% CI
0.1 0.2 0.5 1 2 5 10
Favours no aspiration   Favours aspiration

FIGURE 10.3 Meta-analysis of randomized trials comparing transvaginal aspiration of hydrosalpingeal fluid with no aspiration at the time of oocyte retrieval. Outcome: clinical pregnancy rate.

Sclerotherapy in Conjunction with Transvaginal Aspiration

In an attempt to yield a more permanent effect of transvaginal aspiration, sclerosing agents have been instilled in the aspirated tubes. In a prospective nonrandomised study from China, 33 patients with hydrosalpinx underwent transvaginal aspiration followed by 5–10 minutes of tubal exposure to 98% ethanol, in the cycle prior to starting IVF.[29] No complications occurred, and there was no evidence of recurrence at oocyte retrieval. Pregnancy results were compared with 19 hydrosalpinx patients who had no prophylactic intervention. Implantation and clinical pregnancy rates were significantly higher for patients in the sclerotherapy group, however results were not presented on a per patient basis, but instead per embryo transfer.

A retrospective study has compared interventional ultrasound sclerotherapy to laparoscopic salpingectomy.[30] Although the study was aiming at comparing IVF outcomes, the sample size was too small ($n = 56$) for any valid conclusion regarding effectiveness.

Medical Treatment

The use of antibiotics has been introduced as a simple medical treatment to overcome the negative effects of hydrosalpinx. However, antibiotic treatment has never been prospectively evaluated, and to date, there is only one small retrospective study, which has suggested that extended doxycyclin treatment during an IVF cycle would minimize the detrimental effect of hydrosalpinx.[31]

Other Suggested Management

The use of the natural cycle with the intention to avoid ovarian hyperstimulation and subsequent enlargement of hydrosalpinges has been described in one retrospective study.[32] Patients with hydrosalpinges undergoing IVF in a natural cycle ($n = 72$) demonstrated significantly higher pregnancy rates compared with patients who received controlled ovarian hyperstimulation ($n = 49$) (18% vs. 7%, $p < 0.05$). This result may be biased by the selection of patients to the different treatments. Furthermore, the demonstrated impaired outcome in frozen-thawed cycles contradicts a potential benefit of natural cycles. Any advantage of this method has to be proved in additional studies before it can be considered as an appropriate alternative, taking into account other disadvantages with natural cycles.

The suggestion of increasing the number of replaced embryos to counteract the adverse effect of hydrosalpinges has not been proved effective and should not be considered in times when efforts are made to decrease the rate of multiple pregnancy.

Among all suggested treatment options for hydrosalpinx prior to or in conjunction with IVF, there are only three techniques that have been evaluated in randomized trials. The effect on clinical pregnancy rates of laparoscopic salpingectomy, laparoscopic tubal occlusion and transvaginal aspiration of hydrosalpingeal fluid in comparison with no intervention are summarized in Figure 10.4. All methods proved to be effective, although the estimates for tubal occlusion and transvaginal aspiration are less reliable due to a higher risk of bias in those studies.

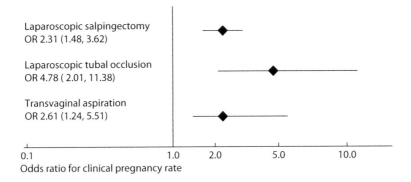

Laparoscopic salpingectomy
OR 2.31 (1.48, 3.62)

Laparoscopic tubal occlusion
OR 4.78 (2.01, 11.38)

Transvaginal aspiration
OR 2.61 (1.24, 5.51)

0.1   1.0   2.0   5.0   10.0
Odds ratio for clinical pregnancy rate

FIGURE 10.4 Meta-analyses of randomized controlled trials comparing surgical intervention with no intervention prior to IVF in patients with uni- or bilateral hydrosalpinges. Common odds ratios and 95% confidence intervals for the outcome clinical pregnancy rate were calculated from data in the Cochrane review and one additional trial. (From Johnson N, van Voorst S, Sowter MC, Strandell A, Mol BWJ. Cochrane Database Syst Rev 2010;(1):CD002125. doi:10.1002/14651858. CD002125.pub3; Fouda UM, Dayed AM. *Gynecol Endocrinol* 2011;27:562–567.)

Impact of IVF on Hydrosalpinx

What happens to the hydrosalpinges when patients undergo IVF? The hydrosalpinges may enlarge during stimulation and may possibly disturb the oocyte retrieval procedure. The hydrosalpinx can be not only accidentally but also intentionally punctured. The risk of infection is described but is not of frequent occurrence. Of greater importance is the case when distally occluded tubes are not detected prior to stimulation, but enlarge and become visible by ultrasound before the aspiration of oocytes. That patient has probably not been informed about the bad prognosis associated with hydrosalpinges, and if the ongoing cycle fails, a discussion of pretreatment directed towards the hydrosalpinx should be initiated.

The sign of endometrial fluid during an IVF cycle has in a few case reports and comparative studies been associated with tubal factor infertility and described as a very poor prognostic sign.[33–35] In two retrospective series including patients with all types of infertility factors, clinical pregnancy rates were significantly impaired if endometrial fluid appeared during ovarian hyperstimulation.[34,35] A summary of studies on effect of endometrial fluid on pregnancy rate is given in Table 10.1. There is no use to aspirate the endometrial fluid prior to transfer because of the rapid recurrence of fluid.[36] Instead, freezing of all embryos and transfer of thawed embryos after salpingectomy should be suggested. Another related clinical symptom is hydrorrhoea, claimed to be associated with poor pregnancy rate after IVF.[33]

Impact of IVF on Hydrosalpinx Treatment

In patients who are surgically treated for their hydrosalpinges, there are a few case reports from which some experience should be acknowledged. Dehiscence at the tubal corners after bilateral salpingectomy has resulted in expulsion of fetuses from

TABLE 10.1

Summary of Studies Comparing the Effect of Endometrial Fluid on the Clinical Pregnancy Rate after IVF

Author Publication Year	Infertility Factor	Endometrial Fluid Present: Pregnancy/Cycle (%)	No Endometrial Fluid: Pregnancy/Cycle (%)	p-Value	Odds Ratio (95% CI)
Andersen 1996	Hydrosalpinx	0/3	7/34 (20.6%)	1.0	–
Levi 2001	All factors (tubal 50%)	15/57 (26.3%)	333/786 (42.4%)	0.02	0.49 (0.26–0.89)
Chien 2002	All factors (tubal 40%)	2/35 (5.7%)	193/711 (27.1%)	0.003	0.16 (0.04–0.68)
Fouda 2011	Aspirated hydrosalpinx	0/2	17/50 (34.0%)	1.0	–

Source: Fouda UM, Dayed AM. *Gynecol Endocrinol* 2011;27:562–567; Andersen AN, Lindhard A, Loft A, et al. *Hum Reprod* 1996; 11:2081–2084; Levi AJ, Segars JH, Miller BT, et al. *Hum Reprod* 2001;16:2610–2615. Chien LW, Au HK, Xiao J, et al. *Hum Reprod* 2002:17:351–356.

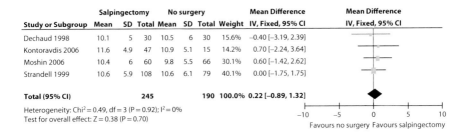

FIGURE 10.5 Effect of salpingectomy on the ovarian reserve measured as number of retrieved oocytes. Meta-analysis of randomized trial comparing salpingectomy with no surgical intervention. Outcome is presented as mean difference in number of oocytes.

the uterine cavity.[37] From this experience, one can learn that the tube should not be excised too close to the uterus. Another report described the adnexal torsion after tubal occlusion for a unilateral hydrosalpinx.[38]

Concern has been raised regarding the potential hazard of disturbing the circulation and innervation to the ovary by performing a radical salpingectomy. Observational studies have shown divergent results when evaluating the number of oocytes retrieved after salpingectomy in comparison with different types of controls. When data from randomised studies are used, and thus more appropriate control groups, there is no difference in the number of oocytes retrieved (Figure 10.5).[18] However, one observational study has demonstrated impairment of the ovarian response, ipsilateral to the salpingectomy after ectopic pregnancy.[39] This finding stresses the importance of a meticulous surgical technique.

Preparing the Patient for IVF

Once a hydrosalpinx has been detected during the infertility workup, by hysterosalpingography (HSG), ultrasound or laparoscopy, careful consideration on further management has to be made. Bearing in mind the poor prognosis without any intervention prior to IVF, information and discussion with the patient are mandatory.

The first step is to evaluate the hydrosalpinx regarding its characteristics. If it is a distally occluded tube with intraluminal adhesions and without any fluid, it can be left without any further interventions. This type of pathology is not suitable for repair and does not affect IVF outcome. In practice, this evaluation can be done by transvaginal ultrasound in most cases, taking into account information from previous examinations.

If prior examination revealed fluid-filled tubes, a discussion on laparoscopic salpingectomy should be initiated with the patient. Psychologically, it is very distressing for the infertile patient to be recommended salpingectomy, in particular if she has bilateral pathology. Bilateral salpingectomy would leave her without any possibility of spontaneous conception and she would have to rely solely on IVF. On the other hand, in the presence of bilateral hydrosalpinges her chances of conceiving and giving birth after IVF are small. The acceptance for salpingectomy is higher in cases of unilateral hydrosalpinx. If the contralateral tube is patent, she may conceive spontaneously, and she has also improved her chances of pregnancy and live birth after IVF.

Pre-IVF Treatment

If the patient with ultrasound-visible hydrosalpinx consents to laparoscopy prior to her first IVF cycle, she should be informed about different possible outcomes such as salpingectomy, tubal occlusion and even salpingostomy. In the ideal situation, the tube can be opened distally and the mucosa inspected and evaluated. If more than half of the mucosa is healthy, the prognosis for spontaneous conception after surgical reconstruction is good.[40] If the interior tube is without any mucosal folds, salpingectomy is the optimal procedure. The original infection causing the hydrosalpinx may also result in adhesions that firmly attach the tube to the peritoneal surfaces and the bowel. The lysis of the hydrosalpinx may carry a high risk of complications with injuries to the adjacent organs, and the salpingectomy procedure may then be replaced by proximal occlusion of the fallopian tube or a smaller tubal resection. Fenestration of the remaining hydrosalpinx may temporarily dispose of the fluid, but the opening reoccludes with the reaccumulation of fluid, which becomes visible by ultrasound.

After salpingectomy or tubal occlusion, it is recommended to wait at least two months for the endometrial environment to restore before starting controlled ovarian hyperstimulation. In the Scandinavian multicenter study, the median time from surgery to embryo transfer was 140 days (range 50–690 days).[15]

Managing the IVF Cycle

Routine stimulation protocols can be applied to hydrosalpinx patients with or without them having undergone any surgical intervention prior to the start. However, it is known that patients with tubal factor infertility may require a higher dose of gonadotrophin, possibly depending on the engagement of the ovary and the subsequent damage from the original infection.

The patient pretreated with salpingectomy can be monitored in the routine program. If tubal occlusion has been performed, the hydrosalpinx will still be visible at sonography and should be recognized during stimulation and puncture avoided at oocyte retrieval. Since communication to the uterine cavity is interrupted, the chance of implantation should not be impaired.

Patients who have not undergone any surgical intervention prior to IVF may require additional ultrasound monitoring to evaluate the enlargement of a previously seen hydrosalpinx or to determine whether previously undetectable tubes have become fluid filled. If hydrosalpinx is visible by ultrasound at the time of oocyte retrieval, transvaginal aspiration of the hydrosalpingeal fluid subsequent to oocyte collection is recommended. Prophylactic antibiotic is mandatory. In cases with bilateral hydrosalpinges, separate needles should be used.

If any endometrial fluid is detected, freezing of all embryos can be considered and transfer postponed until a laparoscopic salpingectomy or tubal occlusion has been carried out.

Patients with previous laparotomies and dense adhesions carry a high risk of complications undergoing laparoscopy, as do patients with obesity. In such cases when laparoscopy is contraindicated, hysteroscopic tubal occlusion by placement of the Essure device can be recommended.

Post-IVF Follow-Up

If the first cycle in patients without any pretreatment for hydrosalpinx does not result in a pregnancy, or a spontaneous abortion occurs, further discussion of salpingectomy or tubal occlusion should be initiated before starting a new cycle.

In the Scandinavian study of salpingectomy, one-third of the patients originally randomized to no intervention prior to their first cycle had a salpingectomy performed after one or two failed cycles. This group achieved the same live birth rate of 55% when cumulative results were calculated, although they had to undergo more cycles compared with the group who had a salpingectomy before their first cycle.

Antenatal controls during pregnancy in patients with hydrosalpinx may draw attention to the possible risk for pelvic infection. Although tubo-ovarian abscesses during pregnancy are rare, cases have been described in which the combination of IVF treatment and hydrosalpinx in patients has been elucidated as a possible risk factor.[41] This risk scenario supports the recommendation of pre-IVF salpingectomy.

Summary of Management Options

Patients with hydrosalpinx have a poor prognosis after IVF and are less likely to conceive and give birth without any pretreatment, compared with patients who have undergone surgical intervention prior to IVF. A treatment protocol is presented in Figure 10.6. Each statement is accompanied by a grade of recommendation based on the evidence level of the reference studies (Table 10.2).[42]

1. Patients with hydrosalpinx large enough to be visible by ultrasound should be recommended laparoscopic salpingectomy prior to IVF, which will double their chance of having a child (evidence level 1a).

2. In cases of severe adhesions to the hydrosalpinx, proximal occlusion of the tube is recommended (level 1a).

3. At laparoscopy, a hydrosalpinx with healthy mucosa can be repaired by salpingostomy and function for spontaneous conception with a fairly good prognosis (level 4).

4. Salpingectomy or tubal occlusion for a unilateral hydrosalpinx increases the chance of spontaneous conception (level 4).

5. Transvaginal aspiration of the hydrosalpingeal fluid at the time of oocyte retrieval should be performed in patients who have not had any surgical pretreatment (level 1a).

6. The presence of endometrial fluid is a poor-prognosis sign, and embryo transfer can be cancelled, embryos frozen and transfer postponed until a laparoscopic salpingectomy has been performed (level 4).

7. Respect should be given to the individual's choice not to undergo salpingectomy due to psychological reasons (level 5).

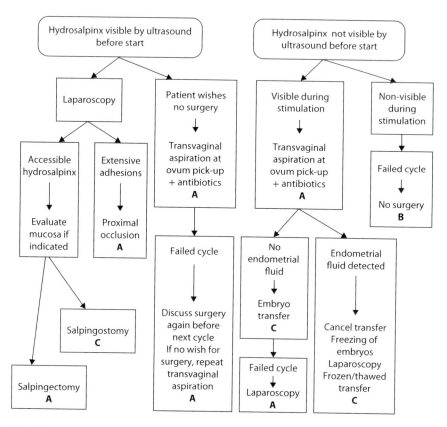

FIGURE 10.6 Treatment protocol for patients with hydrosalpinx undergoing IVF. A–D correspond to grades of recommendation based on evidence levels (Table 10.2). (From Oxford Centre for Evidence Based Medicine. Levels of evidence – March 2009. http://www.cebm.net/?o=1025.)

TABLE 10.2

Strength of Evidence Corresponding to Grade of Recommendation

Level of Evidence	Type of Study/Source	Grade of Recommendation
1a	Systematic review (SR) and meta-analysis with homogeneity of randomised controlled trials (RCTs)	A
1b	Individual RCT (with narrow confidence interval)	A
2a	SR (with homogeneity) of cohort studies	B
2b	Individual cohort study (including low-quality RCT)	B
3a	SR (with homogeneity) of case-control studies	B
3b	Individual case-control study	B
4	Case series (and poor-quality prognostic cohort studies)	C
5	Expert opinion without explicit critical appraisal, or based on physiology, bench research or "first principles"	D

Source: Oxford Centre for Evidence Based Medicine. Levels of evidence – March 2009. http://www.cebm.net/?o=1025.

8. Failure of one cycle should imply a new discussion of salpingectomy or tubal occlusion in order to increase the chance of a live birth (level 1b).

9. To patients in whom laparoscopy is contraindicated, hysteroscopic tubal occlusion by placement of the Essure device can be recommended (level 4).

REFERENCES

1. Strandell A, Waldenström U, Nilsson L, et al. Hydrosalpinx reduces in-vitro fertilization/embryo transfer rates. *Hum Reprod* 1994;9:861–863.
2. Mukherjee T, Copperman AB, McCaffrey C, et al. Hydrosalpinx fluid has embryotoxic effects on murine embryogenesis: A case for prophylactic salpingectomy. *Fertil Steril* 1996;66:851–853.
3. Beyler SA, James KP, Fritz MA, et al. Hydrosalpingeal fluid inhibits in-vitro embryonic development in a murine model. *Hum Reprod* 1997;12:2724–2748.
4. Strandell A, Sjögren A, Bentin-Ley U, et al. Hydrosalpinx fluid does not adversely affect the normal development of human embryos and implantation in vitro. *Hum Reprod* 1998;13:2921–2925.
5. Sawin SW, Loret de Mola JR, Monzon-Bordonaba F, et al. Hydrosalpinx fluid enhances human trophoblast viability and function in vitro: Implications for embryonic implantation in assisted reproduction. *Fertil Steril* 1997;68:65–71.
6. Meyer WR, Castelbaum AJ, Somkuti S, et al. Hydrosalpinges adversely affect markers of endometrial receptivity. *Hum Reprod* 1997;12:1393–1398.
7. Strandell A, Thorburn J, Wallin A. The presence of cytokines and growth factors in hydrosalpingeal fluid. *J Assist Reprod Genet* 2004;21:241–247.
8. Seli E, Kayisli UA, Cakmak H, et al. Removal of hydrosalpinges increases endometrial leukemia inhibitory factor (LIF) expression at the time of implantation window. *Hum Reprod* 2005;20:3012–3017.
9. Daftery GS, Kayisli U, Seli E, et al. Salpingectomy increases peri-implantation endometrial HOXA10 expression in women with hydrosalpinx. *Fertil Steril* 2007;87:367–372.
10. Zeyneloglu HB, Arici A. Olive DL. Adverse effects of hydrosalpinx on pregnancy rates after *in vitro* fertilization-embryo transfer. *Fertil Steril* 1998;70:492–499.
11. Akman MA, Garcia JE, Damewood MD, et al. Hydrosalpinx affects the implantation of previously cryopreserved embryos. *Hum Reprod* 1996;11:1013–1014.
12. Camus E, Poncelet C, Goffinet F, et al. Pregnancy rates after IVF in cases of tubal infertility with and without hydrosalpinx: Meta-analysis of published comparative studies. *Hum Reprod* 1999;14:1243–1249.
13. Freeman MR, Whitworth CM, Hill GA. Permanent impairment of embryo development by hydrosalpinges. *Hum Reprod* 1998;13:983–986.
14. Murray DL, Sagoskin AW, Widra EA, et al. The adverse effect of hydrosalpinges on *in vitro* fertilization pregnancy rates and the benefit of surgical correction. *Fertil Steril* 1998;69:41–45.
15. Strandell A, Lindhard A, Waldenström U, et al. Hydrosalpinx and IVF outcome: a prospective, randomized multicentre trial in Scandinavia on salpingectomy prior to IVF. *Hum Reprod* 1999;14:2762–2769.
16. Wainer R, Camus E, Camier B, et al. Does hydrosalpinx reduce the pregnancy rate following *in vitro* fertilization. *Fertil Steril* 1997;68:1022–1026.
17. deWit W, Gowrising CJ, Kuik DJ, et al. Only hydrosalpinges visible on ultrasound are associated with reduced implantation and pregnancy rates after in-vitro fertilization. *Hum Reprod* 1998;13:1696–1701.

18. Johnson N, van Voorst S, Sowter MC, Strandell A, Mol BWJ. Surgical treatment for tubal disease in women due to undergo *in vitro* fertilisation. *Cochrane Database Syst Rev* 2010;(1):CD002125. doi:10.1002/14651858.CD002125.pub3.

19. Strandell A, Lindhard A, Waldenstrom U, et al. Hydrosalpinx and IVF outcome: Cumulative results after salpingectomy in a randomized controlled trial. *Hum Reprod* 2001;16:2403–2410.

20. Sagoskin AW, Lessey BA, Mottla GL, et al. Salpingectomy or proximal tubal occlusion of unilateral hydrosalpinx increases the potential for spontaneous pregnancy. *Hum Reprod* 2003;18:2634–22637.

21. Kontoravdis A, Makrakis E, Pantos K, et al. Proximal tubal occlusion and salpingectomy results in similar improvement in *in vitro* fertilization outcome in patients with hydrosalpinx. *Fertil Steril* 2006;86:1642–1649.

22. Hitkari JA, Singh SS, Shapiro HM, et al. Essure treatment of hydrosalpinges. *Fertil Steril* 2007;88:1663–1666.

23. Mijatovic V, Dreyer K, Emanuel MH, et al. Essure® hydrosalpinx occlusion prior to IVF-ET as an alternative to laparoscopic salpingectomy. *Eur J Obstet Gynecol Reprod Biol* 2012;161:42–45.

24. Galen DI, Khan N, Richter KS. Essure multicenter off-label treatment for hydrosalpinx before *in vitro* fertilization. *J Minim Invasive Gynecol* 2011;18:338–342.

25. Matorras R, Rabanal A, Prieto B, et al. Hysteroscopic hydrosalpinx occlusion with Essure device in IVF patients when salpingectomy or laparoscopy is contraindicated. *Eur J Obstet Gynecol Reprod Biol* 2013;169:54–59.

26. Darwish AM, El Saman AM. Is there a role for hysteroscopic tubal occlusion of functionless hydrosalpinges prior to IVF/ICSI in modern practice? *Acta Obstet Gynecol* 2007;86:1484–1489.

27. Hammadieh N, Coomarasamy A, Ola B, et al. Ultrasound-guided hydrosalpinx aspiration during oocyte collection improves pregnancy outcome in IVF: A randomized controlled trial. *Hum Reprod* 2008;23:1113–1117.

28. Fouda UM, Sayed AM. Effect of ultrasound-guided aspiration of hydrosalpingeal fluid during oocyte retrieval on the outcomes of *in vitro* fertilization-embryo transfer: A randomised controlled trial. *Gynecol Endocrinol* 2011;27:562–567.

29. Jiang H, Pei H, Zhang W, et al. A prospective clinical study of interventional ultrasound sclerotherapy on women with hydrosalpinx before *in vitro* fertilization and embryo transfer. *Fertil Steril* 2010;94:2854–2856.

30. Na ED, Cha DH, Cho JH, et al. Comparison of IVF-ET outcomes in patients with hydrosalpinx pretreated with either sclerotherapy or laparoscopic salpingectomy. *Clin Exp Reprod Med* 2012;39:182–186.

31. Hurst BS, Tucker KE, Awoniyi CA, et al. Hydrosalpinx treated with extended doxycyclin does not compromise the success of *in vitro* fertilization. *Fertil Steril* 2001;75:1017–1019.

32. Lindheim SR, Hellner D, Ditkoff EC, et al. Ovarian hyperstimulation compounds the deleterious effect of hydrosalpinx on outcome during IVF-ET. *Assist Reprod Rev* 1997;7:64–66.

33. Andersen AN, Lindhard A, Loft A, et al. The infertile patient with hydrosalpinges – IVF with or without salpingectomy. *Hum Reprod* 1996;11:2081–2084.

34. Levi AJ, Segars JH, Miller BT, et al. Endometrial cavity fluid is associated with poor ovarian response and increased cancellation rates in ART cycles. *Hum Reprod* 2001;16:2610–2615.

35. Chien LW, Au HK, Xiao J, et al. Fluid accumulation within the uterine cavity reduces pregnancy rates in women undergoing IVF. *Hum Reprod* 2002;17:351–356.

36. Hinckley MD, Milki AA. Rapid reaccumulation of hydrometra after drainage at embryo transfer in patients with hydrosalpinx. *Fertil Steril* 2003;80:1268–1271.

37. Inovay J, Marton T, Urbancsek J, et al. Spontaneous bilateral cornual uterine dehiscence early in the second trimester after bilateral laparoscopic salpingectomy and in-vitro fertilization: Case report. *Hum Reprod* 1999;14:2471–2473.

38. LaCombe J, Ginsburg F. Adnexal torsion in a patient with hydrosalpinx who underwent tubal occlusion before *in vitro* fertilization. *Fertil Steril* 2003;79:437–438.

39. Lass A, Ellenbogen A, Croucher C, et al. Effect of salpingectomy on ovarian response to superovulation in an *in vitro* fertilization-embryo transfer program. *Fertil Steril* 1998;70:1035–1038.

40. Vasquez HB, Arici A, Olive D, et al. Prospective study of tubal mucosal lesions and fertility in hydrosalpinges. *Hum Reprod* 1995;10:1075–1078.

41. Matsunaga Y, Fukushima K, Nozaki M, et al. A case of pregnancy complicated by the development of a tubo-ovarian abscess following *in vitro* fertilization and embryo transfer. *Am J Perinatol* 2003;20:277–282.

42. Oxford Centre for Evidence Based Medicine. Levels of evidence – March 2009. http://www.cebm.net/?o=1025.

11

The Patient with Endometriosis

Y Cheong

CONTENTS

KEY WORDS: *endometriosis, in vitro fertilisation, assisted conception, pelvic pain, pregnancy*

Background

Endometriosis is a disease whereby endometrial-like tissue exists outside the uterus. The exact prevalence of endometriosis is unknown, although it is estimated that up to 10% of women in the general population and up to 50% of subfertile women have the condition.[1] It is a chronic inflammatory adhesive condition known to be detrimental to fertility. Women with endometriosis may also present with pelvic pain, although severity of pain symptoms may not always reflect accurately on the severity of disease.

Clinically, the accurate diagnosis of endometriosis is fraught with difficulty. The diagnosis of the condition is based on clinical history, examination and imaging of the pelvis (e.g. transvaginal ultrasound) in addition to laparoscopy. Clinically, the presenting symptoms of women with endometriosis overlap significantly with other non-endometriotic gynaecological conditions. Surgically, different appearances of peritoneal endometriosis exist, and these may not always be easily recognisable; intra-operative diagnosis of the condition is often although not always supported by histological confirmation. The disease can be graded in accordance to the American Fertility Score (AFS) system as minimal, mild, moderate or severe,[2] although this classification system has been criticised for not being clinically useful as it does not reflect accurately on pain or subfertility outcomes. Given the variable presentation of this condition, there is almost always a considerable delay in its diagnosis, which clearly contributes to suboptimal care and distress among endometriosis sufferers.[3,4] Research into non-invasive biomarkers[5] and clinical predictive models[6] has not currently yielded highly predictive results thus far.

Endometriosis is a condition of high disease burden.[7] It is a chronic disease akin to diabetes mellitus, requiring multidisciplinary care. It is suggested that care for women with endometriosis be limited to specialised tertiary centres where multidisciplinary input can be streamlined within the patient pathway. However, in reality, the models of care for women with endometriosis vary across the world, and repeat surgeries for these patients due to recurrence of symptoms and/or disease are common occurrences.[8]

A significant number of women with endometriosis will eventually present to the fertility specialist. This chapter provides a critical appraisal of the current evidence in the management of the fertility patient with endometriosis, particularly those seeking treatment using IVF (in vitro fertilisation).

Impact of Endometriosis on IVF and Pregnancy

A poorer reproductive outcome is associated with subfertile women with endometriosis undergoing artificial reproductive treatment (ART).[9–13] A meta-analysis[14] performed over 10 years ago indicated that the pregnancy rate is halved in women with endometriosis undergoing IVF treatment. A more recent meta-analysis[15] examined 27 observational studies involving 8984 women and reported reduced fertilisation rate in stage I/II of endometriosis (relative risk [RR] = 0.93, 95% confidence interval [95% CI] 0.87–0.99, $P = 0.03$), a decrease in the implantation rate (RR = 0.79, 95% CI 0.67–0.93, $P = 0.006$) and clinical pregnancy rate (RR = 0.79, 95% CI 0.69–0.91, $P = 0.0008$) in women with stage III/IV endometriosis undergoing IVF treatment. However, the generalizability of the results of many of these studies, given their non-randomised controlled nature, is limited given the results are significantly confounded. For example, many of these studies did not specify if their included patients had prior surgical or medical treatment, and several had controls with a mixture of non-endometriotic pathologies such as tubal disease. The treatment of women with endometriosis prior to assisted conception, whether medical or surgical, must therefore be individualized.

The exact mechanism whereby endometriosis may detrimentally influence fertility is unknown. Subfertility can be in part attributed to adhesive pelvic disease secondary to the inflammatory nature of the condition resulting in the distortion of the tubo-ovarian anatomy affecting ovum pickup. The peritoneal environment of women with endometriosis is deemed 'hostile' to oocyte and sperm function and development[16–18] and can potentially adversely influence uterine receptivity.

Impact of IVF and Pregnancy on Endometriosis

Controlled ovarian hyperstimulation (COH) used in IVF/ICSI (intra-cytoplasmic sperm injection) treatment leads to the development of multiple follicles and a significant increase in serum oestradiol levels. One of the concerns in women with endometriosis undergoing IVF, given endometriosis is an oestrogen-dependent condition, is the theoretical increased risk of disease progression after COH. While retrospective studies in the 1990s suggested that IVF can potentially dramatically increase one's risk of recurrence of endometriosis,[19] more up-to-date studies suggested the contrary, that IVF does not expose women to consistent risk of progression of endometriosis-related symptoms. However, much of the current evidence is based on short-/intermediate-term outcome data, and long-term follow-up data is still lacking.[20]

Preparing the Patient for IVF

Medical Treatment

In the context of the patient with endometriosis, it is generally recognised that hormonal manipulation, which results in suppression of ovulation, is ineffective in the treatment of subfertility,[21] whether used alone or before and/or after surgery[22] in enhancing pregnancy outcomes. However, treatment with a gonadotrophin-releasing hormone (GnRH) agonist for 3–6 months[23] prior to treatment with IVF increases the odds of clinical pregnancy by more than fourfold.

Surgical Treatment

Surgical intervention is generally thought to be beneficial because it facilitates the removal of diseased endometriotic tissue and helps restore distorted anatomy, although the drawbacks of surgical complications can be significant particularly in those women with ovarian and/or severe disease.[24–26]

Spontaneous Pregnancy

Two multicentre randomised controlled trials (RCTs; $n = 437$) directly addressed the question of whether laparoscopic surgery improved spontaneous pregnancy outcomes in women with unexplained subfertility.[27,28] Both studies compared operative laparoscopic surgery in women with stage I or II endometriosis with diagnostic laparoscopy alone; none of the patients included had severe endometriosis or endometriomas. While Gruppo Italiano in 1999 reported a small negative effect on live births after 12 months, Marcoux et al. in 1997 reported a large positive effect for surgery on ongoing pregnancies. The combined meta-analysis of these two studies showed an advantage of laparoscopic surgery to diagnostic laparoscopy on women with endometriosis (OR 1.64, 95% CI 1.05 to 2.57), although clearly given the conflicting results in the two studies, this result needs to be interpreted with caution. The evidence for the surgical management of severe endometriosis and/or deep infiltrating endometriosis is currently limited. Observational retrospective studies based on small case series suggested that the spontaneous pregnancy rate after surgical treatment of moderate-to-severe endometriosis is between 52% and 69%[29,30] compared to expectant pregnancy rates of 0–33% after expectant management. Prior to proceeding to surgery in the fertility patients seeking to improve their chances of spontaneous conception, the patients will have to be counselled about the potential significant risk of complications related to this type of surgery (total post-operative complication rate of 14%).[31]

Assisted Conception

Given surgical treatment improves spontaneous pregnancy rates in women with minimal and mild endometriosis, it is often extrapolated that surgical treatment should be beneficial to pregnancy outcomes prior to IVF. Only one retrospective study ($n = 661$) has examined this very question.[32] In the group with surgery prior to ART, significantly higher implantation, pregnancy and live birth rates were found. Guidance from the European Society for Human Reproduction and Embryology (ESHRE) working party in 2013 recommended the surgical treatment of AFS/ASRM (American Society for Reproductive Medicine) stage I/II endometriosis prior to IVF, but due to the absence of good evidence, the working party did not provide firm guidance on the preferred surgical management of deep nodular lesions prior to ART.[21] The National Institute of Clinical Excellence in 2013 in contrast suggested that women with moderate or severe endometriosis be offered surgical treatment because it improves the chance of pregnancy, although this guidance is not specific to women undergoing IVF/ICSI.

The benefit of surgical treatment of endometriomas prior to IVF with respect to improving the outcome of IVF is not supported by robust RCTs. The surgical removal of endometriomas may improve access to ovaries and reduce the incidence of post-oocyte retrieval infection, although the surgical treatment itself may damage/decrease the ovarian reserve. A meta-analysis based on the results of 19 observational studies showed that the surgical treatment of endometriomas prior to IVF had no significant effect on IVF pregnancy rates.[33] The only RCT ($n = 99$), not included in the last meta-analysis, comparing the cystectomy versus aspiration of endometrioma, showed some evidence of reduced ovarian response after surgical treatment of endometrioma and lower number of oocytes retrieved.[34] In general, clinicians will consider surgical management of endometriomas greater than 3 cm if they were symptomatic or for the improvement of access to the ovaries.[21]

The optimal management of the woman with endometriosis therefore often presents as a clinical conundrum. Surgery carries not insignificant risks, particularly in women with severe deep infiltrating endometriosis, and thus individualisation of care is crucial; optimal management depends on key fertility determinants such as age, ovarian reserve, symptoms of pain related to the disease, and other surgical co-morbidities such as previous surgery (which may further increase the risk of surgical complications). It may be that in some, the optimal route is for IVF to be attempted first before the consideration of more extensive surgery, while for the more symptomatic patient, surgical management may take precedence. Transvaginal localisation of the ovaries to assess their accessibility for monitoring follicular growth and oocyte retrieval via transvaginal ultrasound scan can also be useful prior to embarking on surgery or IVF.

Complementary Therapy

The potential benefits and harms of complementary and alternative therapy in the context of IVF in women with endometriosis are unclear. This form of therapy cannot be routinely recommended, although many seek these treatments and the potential placebo effect may be high.

Management during IVF Treatment

The optimal management of the patient with endometriosis depends on various factors:

1. The presence of other symptoms of endometriosis other than subfertility (e.g. pelvic pain, dysmenorrhea, dyspareunia, dyschezia)
2. The severity of the endometriosis
3. The presence or absence of endometriomas and their size
4. Key fertility parameters (e.g. ovarian reserve, age, semen analysis)
5. Overall health of the couple (e.g. body mass index [BMI], smoking, alcohol consumption)

A suggested management strategy for the patient who presents with endometriosis is depicted in Figure 11.1. Adequate discussion and counselling should be provided prior to the institution of treatment. If surgery was the first choice of management, the

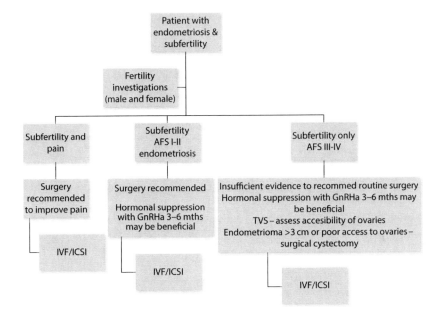

FIGURE 11.1 Management pathway for the patient presenting with endometriosis. AFS, American Fertility Score staging; DIE, deep infiltrating endometriosis; GnRHa, gonadotrophin-releasing hormone analogue; TVS, transvaginal ultrasound scan; > greater.

patient should be informed of the possible risks and benefits of surgery (see previous section on surgical treatment) versus treatment via IVF/ICSI.

Which Stimulation Protocol?

Sallam et al. in 2006 reported, based on the combined results of 3 RCTs, that pre-treatment of women with endometriosis with a GnRHa (gonadotrophin-releasing hormone analogue) for at least 3 months (and up to 6 months) before IVF/ICSI increased the odds of clinical pregnancy fourfold.[35] If GnRHa is used prior to the IVF/ICSI cycle, many will continue the treatment using a long agonist protocol. Indeed, most published data suggest that patients with confirmed endometriosis are treated with the long agonist protocol for the purpose of disease suppression.[36] However, more recent prospective studies have found similar pregnancy rates in women with endometriosis who had undergone GnRH antagonist versus GnRHa IVF/ICSI treatment cycles.[37,38] There are however no RCTs with head-to-head comparisons of the two different treatment regimes specific to women with endometriosis. The ovarian stimulation regime used on women with endometriosis undergoing IVF/ICSI must take into account the centre's individual expertise and the patient's preference. While GnRHa cycles are advantageous in terms of cycle planning, GnRH antagonist cycles are regarded as more patient friendly.[39]

Management in Early Pregnancy

Endometriosis is associated with a range of pregnancy complications, namely spontaneous haemoperitoneum in pregnancy, obstetric haemorrhage, and preterm birth, independent of the assisted reproductive technology. In up to 20% of cases, endometriomas can expand during pregnancy, constituting a risk factor for abscess formation or rupture. Endometriosis implants within the gastrointestinal tract or appendix can perforate. These complications can occur during the antenatal or postnatal period and were only recently acknowledged as a potential major contributor to significant maternal and perinatal mortality and morbidity. The mechanisms around how endometriosis results in many of these complications are still largely unknown, although they are likely to be associated with the invasiveness of the ectopic endometrial implants and the aberrant cellular and molecular integrity of the eutopic endometrium and myometrium, including the junctional zone.[40]

Conclusion

Endometriosis is a disease with many guises. Given that there are unlikely to be any blockbuster drugs on the horizon to eradicate the condition any time soon, clinicians need to base their current management on current best evidence. The presence of endometriosis is detrimental to fertility. To help women who suffer from endometriosis achieve a successful pregnancy, clinicians ought to have considered, in conjunction with the patient and her partner, ideally within the setting of a multidisciplinary team, when and where medical, surgical and/or assisted conception is to be recommended.

REFERENCES

1. Meuleman C, Vandenabeele B, Fieuws S, Spiessens C, Timmerman D, D'Hooghe T. High prevalence of endometriosis in infertile women with normal ovulation and normospermic partners. *Fertility and Sterility* 2009;92(1):68–74.
2. Revised American Fertility Society classification of endometriosis: 1985. *Fertility and Sterility* 1985;43(3):351–2.
3. Stratton P. The tangled web of reasons for the delay in diagnosis of endometriosis in women with chronic pelvic pain: will the suffering end? *Fertility and Sterility* 2006;86(5):1302–4; discussion 17.
4. Nnoaham KE, Hummelshoj L, Webster P, d'Hooghe T, de Cicco Nardone F, de Cicco Nardone C, et al. Impact of endometriosis on quality of life and work productivity: A multicenter study across ten countries. *Fertility and Sterility* 2011;96(2):366–73 e8.
5. Verit FF, Cetin O. Biomarkers of endometriosis. *Fertility and Sterility* 2013;100(4):e19.
6. Nnoaham KE, Hummelshoj L, Kennedy SH, Jenkinson C, Zondervan KT. Developing symptom-based predictive models of endometriosis as a clinical screening tool: Results from a multicenter study. *Fertility and Sterility* 2012;98(3):692–701 e5.
7. Simoens S, Dunselman G, Dirksen C, Hummelshoj L, Bokor A, Brandes I, et al. The burden of endometriosis: Costs and quality of life of women with endometriosis and treated in referral centres. *Human Reproduction* 2012;27(5):1292–9.
8. Guo SW. Recurrence of endometriosis and its control. *Human Reproduction Update* 2009;15(4):441–61.
9. Coccia ME, Rizzello F, Mariani G, Bulletti C, Palagiano A, Scarselli G. Impact of endometriosis on *in vitro* fertilization and embryo transfer cycles in young women: A stage-dependent interference. *Acta Obstetricia et Gynecologica Scandinavica* 2011;90(11):1232–8.
10. Kuivasaari P, Hippelainen M, Anttila M, Heinonen S. Effect of endometriosis on IVF/ICSI outcome: Stage III/IV endometriosis worsens cumulative pregnancy and live-born rates. *Human Reproduction* 2005;20(11):3130–5.
11. Lin XN, Wei ML, Tong XM, Xu WH, Zhou F, Huang QX, et al. Outcome of *in vitro* fertilization in endometriosis-associated infertility: A 5-year database cohort study. *Chinese Medical Journal* 2012;125(15):2688–93.
12. Simon C, Gutierrez A, Vidal A, de los Santos MJ, Tarin JJ, Remohi J, et al. Outcome of patients with endometriosis in assisted reproduction: Results from in-vitro fertilization and oocyte donation. *Human Reproduction* 1994;9(4):725–9.
13. Tummon IS, Colwell KA, Mackinnon CJ, Nisker JA, Yuzpe AA. Abbreviated endometriosis-associated infertility correlates with *in vitro* fertilization success. *Journal of in vitro Fertilization and Embryo Transfer: IVF* 1991;8(3):149–53.
14. Barnhart K, Dunsmoor-Su R, Coutifaris C. Effect of endometriosis on *in vitro* fertilization. *Fertility and Sterility* 2002;77(6):1148–55.
15. Harb H, Gallos I, Chu J, Harb M, Coomarasamy A. The effect of endometriosis on *in vitro* fertilisation outcome: A systematic review and meta-analysis. *BJOG* 2013.
16. Mansour G, Abdelrazik H, Sharma RK, Radwan E, Falcone T, Agarwal A. L-Carnitine supplementation reduces oocyte cytoskeleton damage and embryo apoptosis induced by incubation in peritoneal fluid from patients with endometriosis. *Fertility and Sterility* 2009;91(5 Suppl):2079–86.
17. Mansour G, Aziz N, Sharma R, Falcone T, Goldberg J, Agarwal A. The impact of peritoneal fluid from healthy women and from women with endometriosis on sperm DNA and its relationship to the sperm deformity index. *Fertility and Sterility* 2009;92(1):61–7.

18. Mansour G, Sharma RK, Agarwal A, Falcone T. Endometriosis-induced alterations in mouse metaphase II oocyte microtubules and chromosomal alignment: A possible cause of infertility. *Fertility and Sterility* 2010;94(5):1894–9.
19. Govaerts I, Devreker F, Delbaere A, Revelard P, Englert Y. Short-term medical complications of 1500 oocyte retrievals for *in vitro* fertilization and embryo transfer. *European Journal of Obstetrics, Gynecology, and Reproductive Biology* 1998;77(2):239–43.
20. Benaglia L, Somigliana E, Santi G, Scarduelli C, Ragni G, Fedele L. IVF and endometriosis-related symptom progression: Insights from a prospective study. *Human Reproduction* 2011;26(9):2368–72.
21. Dunselman GA, Vermeulen N, Becker C, Calhaz-Jorge C, D'Hooghe T, De Bie B, Heikinheimo O, Horne AW, Kiesel L, Nap A, Prentice A, Saridogan E, Soriano D, Nelen W. *Human Reproduction* 2014 Mar;29(3):400–12. doi: 10.1093/humrep/det457. Epub 2014 Jan 15.
22. Furness S, Yap C, Farquhar C, Cheong YC. Pre and post-operative medical therapy for endometriosis surgery. *Cochrane Database of Systematic Reviews* 2004(3):CD003678.
23. Sallam HN, Garcia-Velasco JA, Dias S, Arici A. Long-term pituitary down-regulation before *in vitro* fertilization (IVF) for women with endometriosis. *Cochrane Database of Systematic Reviews* 2006(1):CD004635.
24. Somigliana E, Berlanda N, Benaglia L, Vigano P, Vercellini P, Fedele L. Surgical excision of endometriomas and ovarian reserve: A systematic review on serum anti-mullerian hormone level modifications. *Fertility and Sterility* 2012;98(6):1531–8.
25. Carmona F, Chapron C, Martinez-Zamora MA, Santulli P, Rabanal A, Martinez-Florensa M, et al. Ovarian endometrioma but not deep infiltrating endometriosis is associated with increased serum levels of interleukin-8 and interleukin-6. *Journal of Reproductive Immunology* 2012;95(1–2):80–6.
26. Uncu G, Kasapoglu I, Ozerkan K, Seyhan A, Oral Yilmaztepe A, Ata B. Prospective assessment of the impact of endometriomas and their removal on ovarian reserve and determinants of the rate of decline in ovarian reserve. *Human Reproduction* 2013;28(8):2140–5.
27. Marcoux S, Maheux R, Berube S. Laparoscopic surgery in infertile women with minimal or mild endometriosis. Canadian Collaborative Group on Endometriosis. *The New England Journal of Medicine* 1997;337(4):217–22.
28. Italiano G. Prevalence and anatomical distribution of endometriosis in women with selected gynaecological conditions: Results from a multicentric Italian study. Gruppo Italiano per lo Studio dell'Endometriosi. *Human Reproduction* 1994;9(6):1158–62.
29. Stepniewska A, Pomini P, Bruni F, Mereu L, Ruffo G, Ceccaroni M, et al. Laparoscopic treatment of bowel endometriosis in infertile women. *Human Reproduction* 2009;24(7):1619–25.
30. Stepniewska A, Pomini P, Guerriero M, Scioscia M, Ruffo G, Minelli L. Colorectal endometriosis: benefits of long-term follow-up in patients who underwent laparoscopic surgery. *Fertility and Sterility* 2010;93(7):2444–6.
31. Kondo W, Bourdel N, Tamburro S, Cavoli D, Jardon K, Rabischong B, et al. Complications after surgery for deeply infiltrating pelvic endometriosis. *BJOG* 2011;118(3):292–8.
32. Opoien HK, Fedorcsak P, Omland AK, Abyholm T, Bjercke S, Ertzeid G, et al. In vitro fertilization is a successful treatment in endometriosis-associated infertility. *Fertility and Sterility* 2012;97(4):912–8.

33. Tsoumpou I, Kyrgiou M, Gelbaya TA, Nardo LG. The effect of surgical treatment for endometrioma on *in vitro* fertilization outcomes: a systematic review and meta-analysis. *Fertility and Sterility* 2009;92(1):75–87.

34. Nargund G, Cheng WC, Parsons J. The impact of ovarian cystectomy on ovarian response to stimulation during in-vitro fertilization cycles. *Human Reproduction* 1996;11(1):81–3.

35. Sallam HN, Garcia-Velasco JA, Dias S, Arici A. Long-term pituitary down-regulation before *in vitro* fertilization (IVF) for women with endometriosis. *Cochrane Database of Systematic Reviews* 2006(1):CD004635.

36. Ma C, Qiao J, Liu P, Chen G. Ovarian suppression treatment prior to in-vitro fertilization and embryo transfer in Chinese women with stage III or IV endometriosis. *International Journal of Gynaecology and Obstetrics* 2008;100(2):167–70.

37. Pabuccu R, Onalan G, Kaya C. GnRH agonist and antagonist protocols for stage I–II endometriosis and endometrioma in *in vitro* fertilization/intracytoplasmic sperm injection cycles. *Fertility and Sterility* 2007;88(4):832–9.

38. Rodriguez-Purata J, Coroleu B, Tur R, Carrasco B, Rodriguez I, Barri PN. Endometriosis and IVF: Are agonists really better? Analysis of 1180 cycles with the propensity score matching. *Gynecological Endocrinology* 2013;29(9):859–62.

39. Cheong Y, Macklon NS. New concepts in ovarian stimulation. In: Gardner DK, Rizk BRMB, Falcone T, editors. *Human Assisted Reproductive Technology: Future Trends in Laboratory and Clinical Practice.* Cambridge: Cambridge University Press, 2011:54–71.

40. Brosens I, Brosens JJ, Fusi L, Al-Sabbagh M, Kuroda K, Benagiano G. Risks of adverse pregnancy outcome in endometriosis. *Fertility and Sterility* 2012;98(1):30–5.

12

The Patient with Fibroids

Y Khalaf and SK Sunkara

CONTENTS

Introduction

Uterine fibroids are the most common pelvic tumours, occurring in 30% of women over the age of 30 years. The incidence of fibroids increases with age, and they are more common in certain ethnic populations. Twin studies have shown a strong susceptibility to fibroid development, with monozygotic twins twice as likely to develop fibroids compared to dizygotic twins. The prevalence of fibroids reported in literature is frequently underestimated and varies widely due to differences in diagnostic methods, populations studied and study designs. About 32% of fibroids are diagnosed during routine pelvic ultrasound examination and 13% diagnosed incidentally during treatment for a different condition.

Classification of Fibroids

Fibroids are traditionally classified according to their anatomical location and are divided into submucous, intramural (the commonest site) or subserous fibroids. Submucous fibroids (Figure 12.1) are those that distort the uterine cavity and are further divided

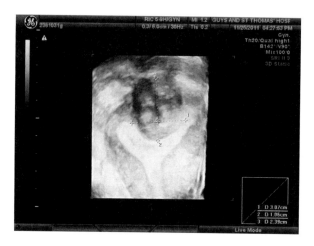

FIGURE 12.1   Three-dimensional ultrasound scan demonstrating a submucous fibroid distorting the fundus of the uterine cavity.

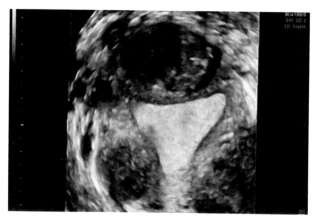

FIGURE 12.2   Three-dimensional ultrasound scan demonstrating an intramural fibroid not distorting the uterine cavity.

into three subtypes: pedunculated (type 0), sessile with <50% intramural extension of the fibroid (type I) and sessile with ≥50% intramural extension (type II). Intramural fibroids (Figure 12.2) are those which do not distort the uterine cavity and with <50% of the tumour protruding into the serosal surface of the uterus. Fibroids protruding ≥50% out of the serosal surface are considered subserosal; they are further divided into sessile or pedunculated. Uterine fibroids are multiple in two-thirds of cases.

Pathogenesis

The underlying pathogenesis and pathophysiology of leiomyomas is highly complex and is far from being completely understood. Cytogenetic examination of leiomyomas reveals that about 40% of them have chromosomal abnormalities.

These consist of translocations, trisomies, deletions and rearrangements. The rest appear chromosomally normal but exhibit mosaicism within the monoclonal tumour. These karyotypic abnormalities have been shown to correlate with fibroid size and site. The mechanisms that link the clinical phenotypes to their underlying genotypes vary. For example, translocations can either upregulate or downregulate a gene and its expressed protein, depending on where the gene sequence is spliced. Trisomies on the other hand generally increase gene expression through increased gene dosing.

Clinical Presentation

The majority of women with fibroids remain asymptomatic. Symptoms associated with fibroids include heavy and prolonged periods, pelvic pressure (from large fibroids), pain (resulting from torsion of a pedunculated fibroid or fibroid degeneration), urinary symptoms and constipation resulting from pressure by anterior and posterior fibroids. Whether fibroids cause infertility is the subject of considerable speculation. Although most women with fibroids are fertile, fibroids may interfere with fertility secondary to anatomical distortion and alterations to the uterine environment. For those women afflicted with fibroids the risks of pregnancy wastage are also increased.

Fibroids and Infertility

While fibroids are associated with infertility in 5–10% of cases, they are estimated to be the sole cause of infertility in 2–3% of cases. The effect of fibroids on fertility is dictated largely by their location and size. The mechanism by which fibroids have a detrimental effect on fertility remains speculative. It has been suggested that fibroids cause infertility by their mechanical nature. Submucous and/or cornual fibroids may directly block the passage of spermatozoa. Fibroids that distort or elongate the endometrial cavity may affect embryo implantation and maintenance of early pregnancy. Submucous fibroids are capable of causing endometrial erosion with subsequent inflammation; they may disrupt the endometrial blood supply, thus affecting implantation and sustenance of the early embryo. It has also been suggested that the hyperoestrogenic environment associated with fibroids may impair fertility.

Fibroids and IVF Treatment Outcome

The advent of assisted reproductive techniques (ARTs) and in particular of *in vitro* fertilisation (IVF) treatment has offered a useful tool to elucidate the relationship between fibroids and fertility. Results from IVF treatment provide precious information on the impact of uterine fibroids on embryo implantation.

There have been meta-analyses that have aimed to assess the impact of fibroids in IVF cycles. Overall, their results showed that fibroids negatively affect pregnancy rates. Although based on a small number of studies, submucous fibroids appeared to strongly interfere with the chance of pregnancy: odds ratio (OR) (95% confidence interval [CI]) for conception and delivery being 0.3 (0.1–0.7) and 0.3 (0.1–0.8), respectively. The adverse impact of intramural fibroids is less dramatic although still significant: OR (95% CI) for conception and delivery being 0.8 (0.6–0.9) and 0.7 (0.5–0.8), respectively.

Evaluation of the location of fibroids on fertility has shown that women with submucous fibroids had significantly lower clinical pregnancy (relative risk [RR] 0.36; 95% CI 0.17–0.73), implantation (RR 0.28; 95% CI 0.12–0.64) and ongoing pregnancy/live birth rates (RR 0.31; 95% CI 0.11–0.85) and a significantly higher miscarriage rate (RR 1.67; 95% CI 1.37–2.05) when compared with infertile women without fibroids. Women with intramural fibroids also had significantly lower clinical pregnancy, implantation and ongoing pregnancy/live birth rates and a significantly higher miscarriage rate. When women with subserous fibroids were compared with women without fibroids, no difference was observed for any outcome measure. It has also been demonstrated that intramural fibroids have an adverse effect on the cumulative live birth rates following IVF treatment.

There had been controversy on the impact of intramural fibroids that do not distort the uterine cavity on IVF treatment outcome. A meta-analysis of 19 studies consisting of a total of 6087 IVF cycles showed a significant decrease in live birth (RR 0.79; 95% CI 0.70–0.88) and clinical pregnancy rates (RR 0.85; 95% CI 0.77–0.94) in women with non-cavity-distorting intramural fibroids compared to those without fibroids. However there is currently lack of evidence from randomised controlled trials whether any intervention in this group of women would improve the outcome of IVF treatment and restore live birth rates to the levels expected in women without fibroids.

Fibroids and Miscarriage

Buttram and Reiter (1981) in their review of published reports from 1957 to 1980 identified a reduction in miscarriage from 41% to 19% in a cohort of women with symptomatic fibroids who underwent myomectomy. Women in these studies had symptomatic palpable fibroids which differ to most infertility patients who have asymptomatic fibroids diagnosed on ultrasound examination. A meta-analysis of controlled studies of intramural fibroids and IVF outcome which reported on spontaneous miscarriage showed a spontaneous miscarriage rate of 22% in women with intramural fibroids compared with 15.4% in the control group. Data to evaluate the risk of miscarriage in women with submucosal fibroids are limited. Casini et al. (2006) reported miscarriages in five of nine (53%) pregnant women with submucosal fibroids and nine of 21 women (43%) who underwent prior myomectomy.

Fertility after Myomectomy

Myomectomy is the preferred surgical treatment option for women wishing to conceive. The procedure may be performed abdominally, laparoscopically or hysteroscopically. Several reviews of literature on pregnancy rates following myomectomy have been published. One of the early reviews focussing on studies published between 1933 and 1980 by Buttram and Reiter (1981) reported a 40% pregnancy rate following abdominal myomectomy (480 of 1202 cases). This rate was 54% when patients with other causes of infertility were excluded. Another review by Vercellini et al. (1998) confirmed this rate of success following myomectomy. They reported a post-surgical pregnancy rate of 57% across prospective studies. When including women with unexplained infertility, this rate was 61%. The advent of endoscopic surgery did not seem to modify this result. In a review by Donnez and Jadoul (2002) the pregnancy rate among women undergoing hysteroscopic and laparoscopic myomectomy was reported as 45% and 49%, respectively. These findings have further been confirmed by more recent and larger studies.

IVF Outcome after Myomectomy

While there is a consistent body of literature on the adverse influence of fibroids on pregnancy outcome, the impact of myomectomy has been less extensively investigated. Narayan and Goswamy (1994) investigated the effect of myomectomy on a small group of women with submucosal fibroids ($n = 27$). They found that the delivery rate was not significantly different in women who underwent myomectomy compared to women without fibroids (37% and 22%, respectively, $P = 0.13$). Surrey et al. (2005) reported a pregnancy rate of 62% and 68%, respectively, in women operated for submucous fibroids and controls without fibroids following IVF treatment. From these studies we can infer that although the overall evidence is scarce, myomectomy did not seem to negatively affect the pregnancy rate following IVF treatment.

A comparative study by Bulletti et al. (2004) has provided further evidence on the effectiveness of myomectomy prior to IVF treatment. Women with intramural and/or subserosal fibroids with at least one lesion >5 cm were allocated to myomectomy or no surgery based on their decision. They reported a live birth rate of 25% and 12%, respectively, in women who did and did not undergo surgery prior to IVF treatment.

Alternative Treatments for Fibroids

Several non-surgical approaches for the treatment of fibroid-associated symptoms have emerged over the last several years with medical therapies as well as radiological interventions being proposed. Gonadotrophin-releasing hormone (GnRH) agonists, the mainstay of medical therapy for fibroids, work by creating a hypogonadotrophic hypogonadal state and produce a significant reduction in uterine size. Their use in the context of infertility treatment remains questionable since ovulation is generally inhibited during treatment and the fibroids usually resume their pre-treatment dimension within a few months after stopping treatment. Other medical options that may reduce the size of fibroids include the androgenic steroid danazol, the antiprogestagen mefipristone, the selective oestrogen receptor modulator raloxifene and the aromatase inhibitor fadrozole. Again because of reasons mentioned their use in the context of infertility treatment remains questionable.

Non-medical alternative treatment options for fibroids that have been developed over the recent past include fibroid embolisation, laparoscopic myolysis and MRI-guided focussed ultrasound. Data regarding pregnancy outcome with these interventions is scanty as most women who wish to conserve fertility have been excluded from these treatments due to safety concerns. Particularly, information on laparoscopic myolysis and MRI-guided focussed ultrasound is absolutely insufficient and the effect of these techniques on pregnancy therefore unknown. Recently, more evidence has been emerging on the effects of fibroid embolisation on pregnancy outcome. In a large survey of 1200 women, Walker and McDowell (2006) recorded 108 women who attempted to become pregnant, of whom 31% were successful. This rate appears to be lower than surgery, but it is difficult to draw definite conclusions as there was no control group. Data regarding pregnancy outcome following uterine artery embolisation tend to support a detrimental effect. An increased risk of miscarriage, preterm delivery, intrauterine growth restriction (IUGR), abnormal placentation and postpartum haemorrhage has been reported. However, these results are controversial, as studies were underpowered. Based on present evidence fibroid embolisation cannot be recommended in daily clinical practice to women wishing to conserve their fertility.

Given the current evidence, clinicians should pursue a comprehensive and personalised approach taking into account the impact of fibroids on fertility, the risks associated with fibroids during pregnancy and the pros and cons of surgery.

A rational approach to addressing fibroids within the context of IVF would be as follows:

1. Submucous fibroids: There is little doubt that submucous fibroids reduce success of IVF treatment by interfering with implantation and increasing the miscarriage rate. It is therefore suggested that such fibroids are resected hysteroscopically prior to IVF treatment.

2. Intramural fibroids:

    a. Symptomatic or asymptomatic intramural fibroids that distort the uterine cavity warrant removal in order to improve symptoms and potentially enhance the outcome of IVF.

    b. Symptomatic or asymptomatic fibroids that do not distort the uterine cavity but are > 4 cm in size have been found in prospective studies to reduce the live birth rate following IVF. Subject to individual cases such fibroids should be removed.

3. Subserous fibroids: These fibroids rarely require treatment as they have little effect on embryo implantation or outcome of IVF. They should be removed only when they are symptomatic or hindering access to the ovaries.

Clinical Scenarios

Patient 1

A 38-year-old woman with an 8-cm intramural/submucous fibroid in the posterior wall of the uterus suffers with menorrhagia and unexplained subfertility. She is not sure whether surgery would help or hinder her fertility and is seeking professional advice.

This woman should be advised to consider having the fibroid removed in order to relieve her menorrhagia and potentially help with her subfertility. Although strong evidence from randomised controlled trials is lacking, there is adequate evidence from observational studies that myomectomy is successful in resolving menorrhagia in 80% of patients. Furthermore, evidence from observational studies has suggested a pregnancy rate as high as 61% over a one-year period following myomectomy in such patients.

Patient 2

A 34-year-old woman considering IVF was found during preparation to have three intramural fibroids (mean diameter between 3 and 4 cm) that were not distorting the uterine cavity. The woman asked for advice regarding whether these fibroids warrant removal before IVF.

This patient should be advised to consider having her fibroids removed surgically before IVF under the following considerations:

1. The available evidence suggests these fibroids may reduce the outcome of IVF treatment.
2. The natural course for fibroids is generally to grow bigger which may aggravate symptoms such as heavy periods.
3. A significant proportion of patients would require surgery anyway within less than 4 years of first diagnosis. It may be appropriate to have the fibroids removed sooner (at a relatively young age) rather than later (>40 years when spontaneous or assisted fertility has significantly declined) so that the potential beneficial impact on IVF outcome would be realised.

REFERENCES

Bulletti C, DE Ziegler D, Levi Setti P, Cicinelli E, Polli V and Stefanetti M. Myomas, pregnancy outcome, and *in vitro* fertilisation. *Ann N Y Acad Sci* 2004;1034:84–92.

Buttram VC Jr, Reiter RC. Uterine leiomyomata: etiology, symptomatology, and management. *Fertil Steril* 1981 Oct;36(4):433–45.

Casini ML1, Rossi F, Agostini R, Unfer V. Effects of the position of fibroids on fertility. *Gynecol Endocrinol* 2006 Feb;22(2):106–9.

Donnez J, Jadoul P. What are the implications of myomas on fertility? A need for a debate? *Hum Reprod* 2002 Jun;17(6):1424–30.

Narayan R and Goswamy RK. Treatment of submucous fibroids and outcome of assisted conception. *J Am Assoc Gynecol Laparosc* 1994;1:307–311.

Surrey ES, Minjarez D, Stevens J and Schoolcraft WB. Effects of myomectomy on the outcome of assisted reproductive technologies. *Fertil Steril* 2005;83:1473–1479.

Vercellini P, Maddalena S, De Giorgi O, Aimi G, and Crosignani PG. Abdominal myomectomy for infertility: A comprehensive review. *Hum Reprod* 1998;13:873–879.

Walker WJ, McDowell SJ. Pregnancy after uterine artery embolization for leiomyomata: a series of 56 completed pregnancies. *Am J Obstet Gynecol* 2006 Nov;195(5):1266–71.

SUGGESTED READING

Klatsky PC, Tran ND, Caughey AB and Fujimotu VY. Fibroids and reproductive outcomes: A systematic literature review from conception to delivery. *Am J Obstet Gynecol* 2008;198:357–366.

Li TC, Mortimer R and Cooke ID. Myomectomy: A retrospective study to examine reproductive performance before and after surgery. *Hum Reprod* 1999;14:1735–1740.

Rackow BW and Arici A. Fibroids and in-vitro fertilisation: Which comes first? *Curr Opin Obstet Gynecol* 2005;17:225–231.

Somigliana E, Vercellini P, Dagauti R, Pasin R, De Giorgi O, and Crosignani PG. Fibroids and female reproduction: A critical analysis of evidence. *Hum Reprod Update* 2007;13:465–476.

Sunkara SK, Khairy M, El-Toukhy T, Khalaf Y, and Coomarasamy A. The effect of intramural fibroids without uterine cavity involvement on the outcome of IVF treatment: A systematic review and meta-analysis. *Hum Reprod* 2010;25:418–429.

13

The Patient with Congenital Uterine Abnormalities

PK Heinonen

CONTENTS

KEY WORDS: *congenital uterine anomalies, Müllerian anomalies, metroplasty, hysteroscopy, assisted reproduction, miscarriage, uterus, preterm, uterine factor infertility*

Background

Abnormal fusion of the Müllerian ducts and failure of absorption of the septum cause varying degrees of congenital uterine malformations ranging from uterine aplasia to a complete double uterus. The etiology of uterine anomalies is unknown but may be multifactorial or polygenic in character. Diethylstilbestrol (DES) exposure in utero is one factor known to cause uterine malformations (T-shaped uterus).

Uterine anomalies have been reported to occur in 5% of the general female population, in 2–3% of fertile women, in 3% of infertile women, and in 5–10% of patients with recurrent miscarriage. Improvement in uterine imaging techniques and especially routine use of transvaginal ultrasound has increased the frequency of their diagnosis. Many uterine anomalies are found incidentally before the first pregnancy.[1]

Congenital uterine malformations are more often associated with poor obstetric performance than with infertility. About 20–25% of patients with uterine anomalies have serious reproductive problems. Recurrent pregnancy wastage, including abortion and premature labor, is the most common clinical manifestation of these disorders, although the majority of such subjects reproduce efficiently.[2]

Uterine malformations are rarely a single cause of primary infertility, except for absence of the uterus or cervical atresia. Primary infertility associated with uterine anomalies may be attributed to related disorders such as endometriosis, pelvic adhesive disease or ovulatory dysfunction. Assisted reproductive treatment is therefore also indicated in some cases with uterine malformations treated by *in vitro* fertilization (IVF). Tubal damage has been the most common etiological factor in assisted reproduction, about half of the patients with uterine anomalies having this background. Unexplained infertility has been found in 6–29% of patients with uterine anomalies treated with IVF.[3,4]

Impact of the Uterine Malformations on IVF and Pregnancy

A number of studies have shown that uterine anomalies are associated with lowered rates of embryo implantation.[4,5] However, in one report of 24 patients with a malformed uterus, implantation rates per embryo transfer (ET) were similar to that in the general infertile population.[3] It is thus possible that other factors such as quality of embryos, number of embryos transferred and technical aspects of the technology of assisted reproduction may affect implantation rates. Surveys published on these topics are so small that conclusions remain invalid.

The classification divides uterine anomalies to the main groups: unicornuate, didelphic, bicornuate, septate and aplastic uterus, although variation between groups is possible.[1] The distribution of these different disorders ranges according to the population, but septate uterus is the most common. The main groups of the uterine malformations are characterized by specific features that determine the prognosis for achieving an ongoing pregnancy and the possible benefits of treatment prior to assisted reproduction. Each main group of anomalies is therefore addressed separately.

Unicornuate Uterus

A unicornuate uterus can be present alone or with a rudimentary horn on the opposite site (Figure 13.1). A non-communicating rudimentary horn is the most common, the communicating type being found rarely. The rudimentary horn may have a cavity, hematometra then being possible. A functional endometrium in the rudimentary horn is rare, but the prevalence of endometriosis is increased compared with other Müllerian anomalies.

A high number of ectopic pregnancies and fetal survival rates of 55–61% have been reported in patients with unicornuate uterus.[1] Most of these patients have only one patent tube adjacent to a functional uterine cavity. Occlusion or removal of this tube means infertility and the need of the assisted reproductive treatment.

Marcus and associates[3] used IVF-ET to treat six (25%) patients with unicornuate uterus out of 24 patients with uterine anomalies, and Heinonen and associates[4] treated eight (47%) of 17 patients. Implantation rates per embryo were 13.2% and 9.6%, and the pregnancy rates per patient were 83% and 75%, respectively. Ectopic pregnancy

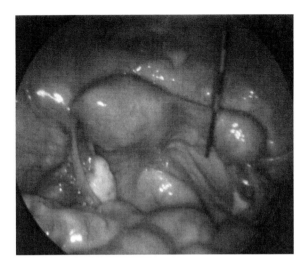

FIGURE 13.1   Unicornuate uterus with rudimentary horn on the right side as seen in laparoscopy.

occurred in three, miscarriage in two, preterm delivery in one and term delivery in five of 11 pregnancies after IVF.[3,4] The unicornuate uterus is associated with a low implantation rate and a risk of ectopic pregnancy in assisted reproductive treatment.

Didelphic Uterus

The didelphic uterine anomaly develops when fusion of the Müllerian ducts is completely lacking, with duplication of corpus and cervix (Figure 13.2). A longitudinal vaginal septum is found in these patients and is mostly the first indication for additional diagnostic procedures.

A didelphic uterus is as common as the unicornuate uterus. Fetal survival rates have been 56–75% in retrospective studies.[6] Only six patients with a didelphic uterus treated with IVF-ET have been reported.[3,4] Marcus and associates[3] had four patients, three of whom delivered after assisted reproduction, and one of these was preterm. Two patients were treated in another study; one of them had a pregnancy after IVF-ET, which ended in miscarriage.[4] Implantation rates per embryo were 27.3% and 6%, respectively.[3,4] The fact that only a few women with a didelphic uterus have been treated with assisted reproduction would imply that infertile patients in this group can be treated mostly by conventional methods, and assisted reproduction is rarely needed. Operative unification of both hemiuteri is not necessary, and this operation should be avoided.

Bicornuate Uterus

Recent endoscopic and imaging diagnostic techniques indicate that many uterine anomalies once considered bicornuate may in fact be septate. The bicornuate uterus is associated with repeated abortion and preterm delivery.[6] Classic abdominal metroplasty according to Strassmann is the recommended therapeutic approach in cases with habitual abortions. This operation is rarely necessary.[1]

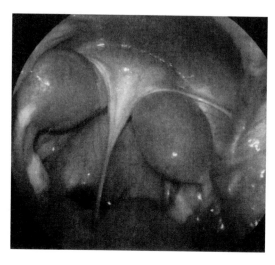

FIGURE 13.2 Laparoscopic view of didelphic uterus. The rectovesical ligament between the hemiuterus is attached anteriorly to the bladder folds between the uteri and attached posteriorly to the serosa of the sigmoid.

Nine patients with a bicornuate uterus treated by IVF have been reported. The implantation rate per embryo was 11.6%, and the pregnancy rate per patient was 44.4%.[3] There were no full-term deliveries among five pregnancies; one was ectopic, one ended in miscarriage and three were preterm deliveries. Guirgis and Shrivastav[7] treated 14 patients with bicornuate uterus by gamete intrafallopian transfer (GIFT); eight (57.1%) achieved a pregnancy after a mean of 2.1 attempts per patient. Assisted reproduction after Strassmann metroplasty of a bicornuate uterus has not been reported.

Septate Uterus

Partial and complete septate uteri are the most common types of uterine anomalies. Transvaginal ultrasound reveals the presence of a uterine septum (Figure 13.3). The anatomy of the uterine septum varies widely, and endoscopic investigations are necessary to exclude a bicornuate uterus.[8] A complete uterine septum sometimes extends through to the cervical canal, and a longitudinal vaginal septum is found.

This anomaly is associated with the poorest reproductive outcome, with low fetal survival rates and a high rate of first-trimester miscarriage.[6,8] Primary infertility is usually not associated with the uterine septum. The indications for assisted reproduction are similar to those without a malformed uterus.

Although there have been no controlled studies to confirm attempts to manage the uterine septum, its treatment seems to improve the prognosis of pregnancy after assisted reproduction.[5,6,9] Lavergne and associates[5] reported 16 cases of septate uterus treated with assisted reproduction. Nine of these women had operative treatment of the uterine septum before IVF-ET, and seven had no treatment. The implantation rate was higher (10.5%) than in untreatable uterine anomalies (4.7%). There were no differences between the groups concerning response to stimulation, quality of

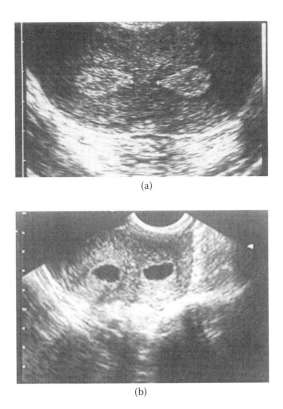

(a)

(b)

FIGURE 13.3 (a) Transvaginal ultrasound shows in transverse scale the septum that divides uterine cavity. (b) Hysterosonography is used to visualize uterine septum and to measure its length and thickness.

embryos or quality of transfers. The authors recommended hysteroscopic treatment of the uterine septum before any attempts at assisted reproduction.[5]

Grimbizis and associates[6] have reported successful results: Eight (72.7%) of 11 patients undergoing hysteroscopic septum resection conceived after assisted reproductive treatment. In another study, seven patients with a subseptate uterus had undergone hysteroscopic incision of the subseptum prior to IVF-ET.[4] The implantation rate per embryo was 8.3%, while the pregnancy rate per embryo was 19.0% and per patient 42.9%. Three of four pregnancies ended in term delivery, and one ectopic pregnancy occurred. These results reflect the situation after surgical repair rather than that in the intact subseptate uterus. One study involved five women with septate uterus and no surgical treatment.[3] The implantation rate was 22.5% and the pregnancy rate per patient 35.7%. Three of five pregnancies ended in first-trimester miscarriages, one had preterm delivery, and only one pregnancy was full term.[3]

Hysteroscopic surgery does not counter infertility, but can improve the prognosis of pregnancy after assisted reproduction. The maturational defects of the septal endometrium found in natural cycles may impair the malformed uterine cavity and prevent reception of the fertilized ovum. Removal of the septum thus not only eliminates an unsuitable site for implantation but also may improve endometrial function.

DES Drug-Related Uterus

Abnormalities such as a T-shaped and hypoplastic uterus have been reported in 70% of DES-exposed women. These patients have had more failures in implantation in an IVF program, in particular in cases of a T-shaped uterus.[2] Hysteroscopic treatment may improve the prognosis of pregnancy. This group is expected to decline in importance as most of these women pass their reproductive years.

Impact of IVF and Pregnancy on Uterine Malformations

The development and availability of assisted reproduction have improved the prognosis for conceiving a pregnancy in some rare uterine abnormalities. For certain anomalies, pregnancy was not possible prior to the era of IVF.

Cervical Atresia

Cervical atresia is an uncommon Müllerian malformation possibly associated with vaginal aplasia. Canalization procedures are performed initially to relieve symptoms related to hematometra and retrograde menstruation.[2] Hysterectomy should be avoided to preserve fertility. The chance of a spontaneous pregnancy is reduced even after successful reconstruction of the genital tract due to severe endometriosis, as well as cervical and tubal factors. Cases of pregnancies after IVF and an ultrasound-guided transmyometrial ET have been published.

Uterine Aplasia

Uterovaginal aplasia is found in 1 per 5,000 females.[2] The condition causes primary infertility. Assisted reproduction has been reported in such women. Surrogate women have been used to transfer the embryo, and results have been comparable to those with conventional IVF. The pregnancy rate per ET was 21.4%, and the pregnancy rate per patient was 50% when six patients were treated with gestational surrogacy. Congenital absence of the uterus and vagina is not inherited in a dominant fashion according to one study of 32 women with Müllerian agenesis undergoing IVF with subsequent ET to a surrogate uterus. IVF surrogacy is controversial and is not accepted in some countries. Uterine transplantation from a mother to her daughter or from a multiorgan donor is a future possibility to treat infertility of women with congenital uterine aplasia.[10]

Preparing the Patient for IVF

Accurate diagnosis of the malformed uterus is necessary prior to assisted reproduction and preparation of the patient for IVF.

Transvaginal ultrasound, hysterosonography and hysteroscopy are used as first-line diagnostic tools. These constitute adequate means to diagnose septate and didelphic uterus. They are not always adequate to detect a rudimentary horn associated with a unicornuate uterus or to confirm a bicornuate uterus. Three-dimensional ultrasound and magnetic resonance imaging (MRI) are more accurate techniques for detection of the anomaly.

Endometriosis is frequently associated with many uterine anomalies, and its laparoscopic treatment before assisted reproduction is recommended. A rudimentary horn associated with a unicornuate uterus has been reported to be associated with endometriosis in 50%. Removal of the rudimentary uterine horn may improve the chances of a successful pregnancy.

A longitudinal vaginal septum is found in women with a complete septate and didelphic uterus. It is mostly asymptomatic. Its incision may facilitate ET in that visualization of the uterine cervix is improved.

Ultrasound scanning of the kidneys is important, as renal malformations are found in 15–25% of women with uterine anomalies. Unilateral renal agenesis is the most common renal anomaly and is associated with the unicornuate and didelphic uterus.

Many authors recommend hysteroscopic incision of a uterine septum prior to assisted reproduction treatment.[4–6] Ban-Frangež and associates[9] reported that hysteroscopic resection of both small and large septum improved prognosis of pregnancy in women treated postoperatively with assisted reproduction. Hysteroscopic incision of the uterine septum is a fairly simple and safe procedure involving low morbidity. Excessively radical incision may damage the uterine muscular wall and incur a risk of rupture of the uterus during pregnancy. A septal remnant less than 1 cm is as good as complete septal incision.

Management during IVF Treatment

Ovarian stimulation, cycle monitoring by serial ultrasound scanning, sperm preparation and embryo culture are standard IVF methods and do not differ in patients with uterine anomalies. Intracytoplasmic sperm injection (ICSI) has been used in cases with low or failed fertilization in conventional IVF or primary male factor.[4]

A unicornuate uterus may be associated with an undescended ovary. This is worthy of consideration when follicles are aspirated after ovarian stimulation in patients with this uterine anomaly.

Embryo transfer is preferably made to the hemiuterus that shows a more suitable endometrium according to ultrasound scanning in patients with a didelphic or complete bicornuate uterus. The cavity of the hemiuterus is often directed markedly laterally, and this may hinder the gentle direction of the transfer catheter into the uterine cavity. Ultrasound is useful in estimating the location of the cavity. Pregnancy has been located more commonly (76%) in the right hemiuterus than in the left.

Many of the published studies in the field cover the period when three embryos were normally transferred, with the concomitant increased risk of multiple pregnancy. Among 24 women with uterine malformations, the multiple pregnancy rate in the group of patients who had three embryos transferred was 40% compared with 0% in those receiving one or two embryos.[3]

In current practice, single-embryo transfer is recommended to reduce the risk of multiple pregnancy and thus the combined risks of a malformed uterus and multiple pregnancy. Although twin pregnancies, even triplets, have been described in malformed uteri, both are risk factors for preterm labor, and using single-embryo

TABLE 13.1

Main Options in Patients with Uterine Malformations Before, During and After Assisted Reproductive Treatment (ART)

Uterine Anomaly	Process	Impact
Before ART		
All	Ultrasound, endoscopies, MRI	To make a precise diagnosis of the malformed uterus
All	Laparoscopic treatment of endometriosis	To provide better outcome of assisted reproduction
Unicornuate	Removal of rudimentary horn	To improve prognosis of pregnancy
Didelphic, septate	Incision of vaginal septum	To facilitate embryo transfer
Subseptate-septate	Incision of uterine septum	To improve implantation rate and prognosis of pregnancy
All	Ultrasound, pyelography	To detect renal anomalies
During ART		
Unicornuate	Oocyte retrieval	Undescended ovaries make it difficult
Didelphic, bicornuate	Embryo transfer	ET to better hemiuterus
All	Embryo transfer	Only 1 embryo
After ART		
Unicornuate	Transvaginal ultrasound	Risk of ectopic pregnancy
Septate	Ultrasound	Risk of first-trimester abortion
All	Ultrasound: measurement of endocervix	Cervical incompetence (cervical cerclage)
All	Ultrasound	Fetal malpresentation, caesarean section
Solitary kidney	Ultrasound, pre-eclampsia investigation	Risk of pre-eclampsia

Note: ET, embryo transfer; MRI, magnetic resonance imaging.

transfer it is possible to reduce these risks. Transfer of cryopreserved-thawed embryos is effected during natural cycles or after artificial hormonal endometrial preparation.

Table 13.1 summarizes some of the options that may be involved in assisted reproductive treatment of patients with uterine anomalies.

Management during Pregnancy

If pregnancy follows assisted reproductive treatment in a malformed uterus, it needs meticulous follow-up. This pregnancy carries at least the same risks as in cases of conception during the normal cycle. It is of prime importance to confirm the site of pregnancy using transvaginal ultrasound (Figure 13.4). Ectopic pregnancy has been reported in all types of malformed uterus after IVF but is most common in women with a unicornuate uterus. First-trimester abortions are associated with a septate uterus, but incision of the septum prior to assisted reproduction improves the prognosis of pregnancy.[5,9]

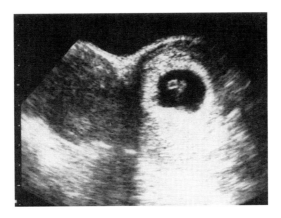

FIGURE 13.4   Transvaginal ultrasound of didelphic uterus with pregnancy in patient's left uterus.

Preterm delivery has occurred in 15–45% of all deliveries in women with a malformed uterus.[1,6] Pregnancy after assisted reproduction also carries a risk of preterm delivery, even in a single pregnancy in a normal uterine cavity. Thus, both factors may increase the number of preterm deliveries.

Prophylactic cervical cerclage has been used in women with uterine anomalies to prevent preterm delivery.[1] The relevant data are mostly from retrospective studies. Patients who have had second-trimester miscarriage or extremely preterm delivery may benefit from the application of cervical cerclage. Transvaginal ultrasound is useful in assessing the length of the cervical canal and the appropriate point of the application.

Unilateral renal agenesis predisposes women with uterine anomalies to gestational hypertension and pre-eclampsia. The condition is often mild but may indicate treatment and delivery earlier than planned.

The caesarean section rates in patients with uterine anomalies delivered after assisted reproduction have been 60–75%.[3,4,7] This is attributed to prematurity and fetal malpresentations, and also a history of infertility may have lowered the threshold for intervention. High frequencies of breech presentation and caesarean section are associated with malformed uteri. Normal vaginal delivery is possible after hysteroscopic incision of a uterine septum.

REFERENCES

1. Rackow BW, Arici A. Reproductive performance of women with Müllerian anomalies. *Curr Opin Obstet Gynecol* 2007;19:229–37.
2. Lin PC, Bhatnagar KP, Nettleton GS, et al. Female genital anomalies affecting reproduction. *Fertil Steril* 2002;78:899–915.
3. Marcus S, Al-Shawaf T, Brinsden P. The obstetric outcome of *in vitro* fertilization and embryo transfer in women with congenital uterine malformation. *Am J Obstet Gynecol* 1996;175:85–9.
4. Heinonen PK, Kuismanen K, Ashorn R. Assisted reproduction in women with uterine anomalies. *Eur J Obstet Gynecol Reprod Biol* 2000;89:181–4.
5. Lavergne N, Aristizabal J, Zarka V, et al. Uterine anomalies and *in vitro* fertilization: What are the results? *Eur J Obstet Gynecol Reprod Biol* 1996;68:29–34.

6. Grimbizis GF, Camus M, Tarlatzis BC, et al. Clinical implications of uterine malformations and hysteroscopic treatment results. *Hum Reprod Update* 2001;7:161–74.
7. Guirgis RR, Shrivastav P. Gamete intrafallopian transfer (GIFT) in women with bicornuate uteri. *J In Vitro Fert Embryo Transf* 1990;7:283–4.
8. Homer HA, Li T-C, Cooke ID. The septate uterus: A review of management and reproductive outcome. *Fertil Steril* 2000;73:1–14.
9. Ban-Frangež H, Tomaževič T, Virant-Klun I, et al. The outcome of singleton pregnancies after IVF/ICSI in women before and after hysteroscopic resection of a uterine septum compared to normal controls. *Eur J Obstet Gynecol Reprod Biol* 2009;146:184–7.
10. Brännström M, Diaz-Garcia C, Hanafy A, et al. Uterus transplantation: Animal research and human possibilities. *Fertil Steril* 2012;97:1269–76.

14

The Patient with Malignant Disease

RA Anderson

CONTENTS

KEY WORDS: *cancer, cryopreservation, IVF, oocyte, fertilization*

Introduction

Patients with cancer present particular challenges to the *in vitro* fertilization (IVF) unit. Many will be struggling to deal with the new diagnosis and may be unwell with their underlying disease. A second group will be cancer survivors, for whom the issues will be more focused on assessment of the impact of their cancer treatment on their fertility. Some of this group will also have concerns about the potential effect of IVF and subsequent pregnancy on their cancer, for example those women with breast cancer.

Cancer is diagnosed in approximately 650,000 women each year in the United States.[1] As treatment of previously fatal diseases such as the acute leukemias has improved, so has the number of young women survivors, whose fertility may have been compromised in a number of ways. The adverse effects of many chemotherapy agents on the ovary have long been recognized,[2] but there is also a considerable prevalence of subfertility in female cancer survivors who retain ovarian function.[3,4] Increasing recognition of the adverse effects of cancer treatment on fertility of both men and women together with this increasing survival has shifted emphasis from treatment and cure at any cost to a greater interest in 'late effects', which includes the preservation of fertility. Patients of both sexes may therefore be referred to IVF units for discussion of the implications of their cancer treatment on their fertility and for consideration of ways to ameliorate any adverse effects. Such patients are of an increasingly wide age range and now include the prepubertal, generating fresh challenges for their caregivers. Approximately 1 in 5000 adolescents are affected with cancer, with an overall cure rate of 75%.[5,6]

This chapter particularly addresses issues relating to the adult patient newly diagnosed with cancer and considering IVF as a means of fertility preservation, including longer-term issues that should be considered during initial assessment and treatment.

Impact of Malignant Disease on Fertility and IVF

Patients with malignant disease may have reduced fertility as a result of their condition. This has long been recognized for men, with approximately 70% of men with Hodgkin's disease having impaired semen quality.[7] Infrequent ejaculation as a result of illness (e.g. pyrexia), anxiety and loss of sexual interest may contribute to this. A possible adverse effect of reduced sexual activity with a prolonged ejaculatory interval should be taken into consideration in assessment of the healthy male partner of the cancer patient. Non-reproductive effects of cancer such as cachexia and fever may also influence female fertility, and this has now been directly assessed (although data can only be compared to a contemporaneous infertile cohort, thus there are opportunities for bias). Initial studies suggested that women with cancer had a reduction in oocyte quality and fertilization rates[8]; a recent meta-analysis confirmed that oocyte number recovered after stimulation was slightly lower in cancer patients (9.0 ± 6.5 vs. 10.8 ± 6.7)[9]; fertilization rates were similar to controls. The proportion of poor responders was also slightly increased (7.8% vs. 5.9%), but this did not reach statistical significance. Insufficient data are available to clarify if particular conditions are associated with reduced ovarian function: Women with Hodgkin and non-Hodgkin lymphoma have been reported to have lower anti-Müllerian hormone (AMH) concentrations than controls,[10] as have younger women with breast cancer.[11] The recovery of fewer oocytes than controls suggests that there may well be an effect of cancer disease processes on the ovary analogous to that long recognized on spermatogenesis, but that this can be largely overcome by gonadotrophin stimulation. The appropriateness of the control group selected is of importance in these assessments as the use of more methodologically robust longitudinal or randomization designs is inappropriate.

Men and women newly diagnosed with cancer and wishing to have children have markedly different options. Cryopreservation of semen, despite the caveats regarding quality mentioned, is now routinely considered and widely available, although there is often little time available between diagnosis, referral to a storage center and the need to initiate treatment. The risk of loss of fertility will be related to the treatment proposed, but the relative ease of semen cryostorage means it is much better to store unnecessarily (and potentially discard later) than miss the opportunity. Patients will be faced with the need to consider the fate of any stored samples in the event of their death; this may be distressing, as patients may have been unwilling or unable to face the reality of their condition prior to that point. Competence to give consent will need to be assessed in adolescent patients.[12] Staff at the storage centre may not have appropriate experience, and this issue should be specifically addressed by the pediatric oncology team before referral. Age-specific patient information can be of great value under such circumstances. Subsequent usage of cryopreserved sperm will be determined by couple-specific factors as in any couple seeking fertility treatment, but with due attention to both the spermatogenic function of the man at that time (which may have recovered to normal) and the quality and quantity of the stored samples, which will inform decision-making as to the appropriate treatment modality. Only approximately 10–25% of men who store sperm under these conditions subsequently use it.[13,14]

If chemotherapy has already been started, consideration should be given as to whether semen storage is still appropriate; it is generally thought not to be, on the basis of animal data showing significant adverse effects on progeny from the use of sperm exposed to chemotherapeutic agents.

Women have no equivalent non-invasive option for fertility preservation. Potential options that should be discussed with the woman and her partner, if any, include taking no specific action, urgent IVF with embryo cryopreservation, oocyte cryopreservation or ovarian tissue cryopreservation. The last is outside of the remit of this chapter but is the subject of considerable recent advances and comprehensive review.[15]

The need to consider urgent IVF will be in part determined by the treatment the woman is about to undergo, as the invasiveness of the procedure and the inherent delay change the basis for decision-making, compared with semen cryostorage. The option to do nothing should be explored, bearing in mind the patient's age, diagnosis and prognosis, and proposed treatment. The option for future use of donated oocytes as an established treatment should be clearly explained. It should also be made clear that there is considerable interindividual variability in the gonadotoxic effects of different anticancer regimens, making accurate estimates of the risk of, for example, premature ovarian insufficiency, difficult. In general, alkylating agent-based chemotherapy (e.g. cyclophosphamide, chlorambucil and busulfan) is markedly more gonadotoxic than that using agents such as doxorubicin and cisplatin, while methotrexate, vincristine and bleomycin have low gonadotoxicity. Alkylating agents are, however, widely used in the treatment of conditions such as breast cancer, leukemia and lymphoma, which are the commoner malignancies of the relevant age group. Oncologists are increasingly using regimens without alkylating agents in lymphoma, such as the ABVD regimen of doxorubicin (adriamycin), bleomycin, vinblastine and dacarbazine), with reduced gonadotoxicity, but there is the risk of cardiotoxicity with anthracycline agents. However, it should be recognized that there may be no dose of agents such as cyclophosphamide that is not toxic to the follicle, with the age of menopause being more subtly influenced at low doses and such patients being at risk of premature ovarian insufficiency even if regular menstruation is resumed.

Radiotherapy not only is very damaging to the ovary[16] but also can have adverse effects on other parts of the reproductive axis, including the hypothalamus, pituitary and uterus. This is of importance to the patient considering IVF, as total body or local irradiation may damage the uterus, resulting in increased risk of miscarriage, premature delivery and low birth weight.[17,18] Multiple pregnancy is therefore a particular risk in these women, and planned single-embryo transfer should be the norm.

IVF requires sperm, so further difficulties arise with the need for a male partner. The existence of a long-term relationship does not necessarily imply that the man wishes to have children with the woman, but he may be under considerable pressure, not necessarily expressed, to be part of the treatment. The necessary raising of the issue may lead to relationship difficulties, and the need for support for both partners should be considered and readily available. The use of donated sperm may be appropriate. Semen analysis may reveal hitherto undetected reproductive dysfunction, with implications for both the immediate treatment cycle and his future fertility. He will need to give his explicit consent for the use of his sperm, and both will need to consider the fate of the embryos in the event of death of either partner, although this will be predominantly directed towards the female cancer patient. Should the woman not have a (male) partner, some of these issues are in fact simplified by the need to use donated sperm.

An alternative option is oocyte cryopreservation, which avoids issues surrounding fertilization. Live birth following this procedure was first reported in 1986, and while initial success rates were modest, the advent of vitrification has had a very substantial impact. Randomised studies have now shown that vitrified oocytes have a similar developmental potential to fresh oocytes[19]; thus this is now undoubtedly the cryopreservation method of choice. This makes oocyte cryostorage a viable option for single women with cancer and gives the further option to those in a relationship of dividing the cohort of recovered oocytes, with vitrification of some directly, and fertilization of others with embryo storage. The longer-term outcomes of such strategies (relating to gamete use and pregnancy) have not however been reported.

There may be issues specific to particular diagnoses. One example is the patient with cervical cancer. Transvaginal oocyte aspiration following ovarian stimulation may not be appropriate because of the risk of bleeding from the tumor, and transabdominal aspiration may need to be considered. Conservative fertility-sparing surgery such as radical trachelectomy may be feasible in some centres for selected patients and may be more appropriate than IVF; experience of fertility in these patients is growing.[20]

Impact of IVF on Malignant Disease

The main concerns regarding whether IVF will impact adversely on the patient with cancer relate to the potential delay in starting the patient's treatment (e.g. chemotherapy) or any possible effects of the hormonal changes on the disease.

Breast cancer is the most common malignant disease in women of reproductive age, and approximately 15% of breast cancer occurs in women under the age of 40. There may be time to perform IVF with embryo or oocyte cryopreservation. Superovulation exposes the patient to high estradiol concentrations, if only for a few days. While the magnitude of the risk over such a short period of time is unclear, understandably however women with estrogen-receptor-positive breast cancers may well wish to avoid even the possibility of such a risk. The use of an antiestrogen such as tamoxifen, widely employed in the treatment of breast cancer, was initially suggested for ovarian stimulation.[21] As an estrogen receptor antagonist, serum estradiol concentrations are not affected, but their action is prevented. Tamoxifen use in IVF regimens can result in reduced gonadotrophin requirements and maintained oocyte numbers, with satisfactory fertilization rates. More recently the use of aromatase inhibitors, particularly letrozole, has also been described in this context.[22,23] This reduces estrogen production markedly, but with maintenance of oocyte yield and with normal fertilization rates, and results in an average of a modest 38 days between breast cancer surgery and starting chemotherapy. The low estrogen production needs to be recognized as no longer being of value in monitoring the ovarian response, particularly important in assessing risk of ovarian hyperstimulation. Such endocrine manipulations may not be necessary in breast cancers not expressing estrogen receptors. Follow-up data indicate that letrozole-based IVF does not alter the risk of breast cancer recurrence, although the number of women studied was limited.[24] In the less common situation of a woman with endometrial cancer, tamoxifen is contraindicated due to its stimulatory effects on the endometrium, but aromatase inhibitors can be used.[25]

Some delay is inevitable, and its impact and magnitude should be discussed with the patient and her oncologist. Considerations for planning the treatment cycle include usual factors such as the patient's normal menstrual cycle, but she may also be using hormonal contraception. Oral contraception is of little consequence and frequently is used to regulate menstrual cycles prior to IVF. The use of depot medroxyprogesterone acetate results in significant hypogonadotropic hypogonadism (i.e. the patient is already down-regulated), but this will be overcome by the administration of exogenous gonadotropins, and its suppressive effects on the endometrium are irrelevant in this context as all embryos will be cryopreserved. The use of gonadotropin-releasing hormone (GnRH) antagonists is probably the most effective way to shorten the IVF cycle if that is of paramount importance and is discussed further later in this chapter.

Preparing the Patient for IVF

For the woman with newly diagnosed malignancy, it is of prime importance that the patient has adequate time to consider whether she (and her partner) wish to proceed with IVF, despite the urgency of the situation. Factors to consider include potential family pressures, relationship issues as well as issues relating to her specific diagnosis, staging and the treatment planned, as well as likelihood of survival. The need for adequate time to consider her options is essential, yet clearly limited. Independent counselling will be invaluable in some cases. Issues regarding the welfare of the child that IVF is being undertaken to create should be considered in the context of long-term prognosis.

Specific pretreatment investigations should be considered in women undergoing IVF who have been treated for cancer in the past. Assessment of the ovarian reserve, by ultrasound measurement of antral follicle count (AFC) or AMH according to clinic practice is particularly important if the woman has previously received any chemotherapy (thus normally in the context of disease recurrence rather than initial diagnosis). Even limited gonadotoxicity may have been significantly deleterious in a woman with an already modest ovarian reserve from being at the lower extreme of normal biological variation. Measurement of AMH has also been demonstrated to be of value in predicting post-chemotherapy ovarian function in women with breast cancer[26] and thus may help shape opinions as to the need for fertility preservation.

Managing the IVF Cycle

The key issues to be considered in planning an 'emergency' IVF cycle are timing, duration (i.e. delay) and safety. The use of GnRH antagonist protocols instead of a long down-regulation cycle has been widely adopted in this context, avoiding the time-consuming need for luteal-phase commencement of down-regulation, and also associated with lower risk of ovarian hyperstimulation. In an initial report of the use of GnRH antagonist in cancer patients, which included pre-stimulation administration of a larger dose (1 mg) for luteolysis when necessary, the median duration of treatment was 12 days.[27] An early follicular start may not be necessary: luteal-phase starting has also been described, and more recently 'random-phase' starting has been demonstrated to be effective. Compared to a non-cancer conventionally treated cohort, a random start resulted in a similar number of oocytes recovered, with good fertilization rates.[28] Treatment duration was 2 days longer than with conventional cycle planning, probably reflecting the absence of the endogenous inter-cycle follicle-stimulating hormone (FSH) rise when treatment is started out with the early follicular phase. One caveat is that pregnancy rate and live birth data are not yet available due to the evolving nature of the field. Asynchrony of the endometrium is not relevant, as all embryos will be cryopreserved in these patients.

The third consideration is safety. The use of letrozole during ovarian stimulation has been mentioned and can be combined with a GnRH antagonist random start protocol.[28] In addition to the relatively short duration of GnRH antagonist cycles, they have the important feature of reducing the risk of ovarian hyperstimulation syndrome (OHSS),[29] which might otherwise add further delay in starting chemotherapy.

Post-IVF Follow-Up

Many patients having IVF under these circumstances will move on to their definitive treatment rapidly after embryo or oocyte cryopreservation and will therefore often not be clinically followed up by the IVF centre. Clearly, it is essential to ensure that no immediate adverse effects have occurred, and this can be achieved by telephone contact. Similarly, the patient should be informed as to the final outcome of treatment and provided with a written record of the number of embryos or oocytes stored. It may be valuable for this written record to restate the conditions of storage (e.g. time limitations), as such considerations may well have been forgotten or not clearly discussed or appreciated during the information overload experienced by these women in the lead-up to treatment.

Some patients will not survive their disease, and it is much more appropriate that this be detected by regular follow-up, for example by annual contact with the patient, their primary-care physician or the physician caring for their malignancy, than only some years after death. Formal systems should be in place for this not to be missed while avoiding insensitive approaches to a bereaved family. Issues surrounding posthumous use or destruction of cryopreserved embryos will have been covered pretreatment, and it may be appropriate for the treatment summary letter or equivalent document to detail this. These and the above issues are summarized in Table 14.1.

TABLE 14.1

Summary of Principal Treatment Considerations

Newly diagnosed malignancy

Assessment of impact of proposed treatment on fertility

Assessment of impact of disease on patient's current health and gonadal function

Consideration of prognosis for patient and consequences of patient's death

Assessment of involvement of partner

Issues over timing of start of IVF cycle in relation to menses/hormonal contraception use

Impact of specific diagnosis

Breast, endometrial, cervical cancer

Influence on treatment cycle

Use of GnRH antagonist, aromatase inhibitor

Risks to patient of IVF treatment

OHSS

Specific issues such as thrombocytopenia, neutropenia

Previously treated malignancy

Assessment of ovarian compromise

   AMH, AFC measurement

Assessment of uterine function if post-radiotherapy

Risk of relapse/long-term survival

Note: AFC, antral follicle count; AMH, anti-Müllerian hormone; GnRH, gonadotropin-releasing hormone; IVF, in vitro fertilization; OHSS, ovarian hyperstimulation syndrome.

REFERENCES

1. Weir HK, Thun MJ, Hankey BF, et al. Annual report to the nation on the status of cancer, 1975–2000, featuring the uses of surveillance data for cancer prevention and control. *J Natl Cancer Inst* 2003; 95: 1276–99.
2. Meirow D, Biederman H, Anderson RA, Wallace WHB. Toxicity of chemotherapy and radiation on female reproduction. *Clin Obstet Gynecol* 2010; 53(4): 727–39.
3. Letourneau JM, Ebbel EE, Katz PP, et al. Acute ovarian failure underestimates age-specific reproductive impairment for young women undergoing chemotherapy for cancer. *Cancer* 2012; 118: 1933–9.
4. Anderson RA. Infertility in women after childhood cancer. *Lancet Oncol* 2013; 14(9): 797–8.
5. Mertens AC, Yasui Y, Neglia JP, et al. Late mortality experience in five-year survivors of childhood and adolescent cancer: The Childhood Cancer Survivor Study. *J Clin Oncol* 2001; 19(13): 3163–72.
6. Wallace WH, Thompson L, Anderson RA. Long term follow-up of survivors of childhood cancer: Summary of updated SIGN guidance. *BMJ* 2013; 346: f1190.
7. Rueffer U, Breuer K, Josting A, et al. Male gonadal dysfunction in patients with Hodgkin's disease prior to treatment. *Ann Oncol* 2001; 12: 1307–11.
8. Pal L, Leykin L, Schifren JL, et al. Malignancy may adversely influence the quality and behaviour of oocytes. *Hum Reprod* 1998; 13: 1837–40.
9. Friedler S, Koc O, Gidoni Y, Raziel A, Ron-El R. Ovarian response to stimulation for fertility preservation in women with malignant disease: A systematic review and meta-analysis. *Fertil Steril* 2012; 97(1): 125–33.

10. Lawrenz B, Fehm T, von Wolff M, et al. Reduced pretreatment ovarian reserve in premenopausal female patients with Hodgkin lymphoma or non-Hodgkin-lymphoma – evaluation by using antimullerian hormone and retrieved oocytes. *Fertil Steril* 2012; 98(1): 141–4.

11. Su HI, Flatt SW, Natarajan L, DeMichele A, Steiner AZ. Impact of breast cancer on anti-mullerian hormone levels in young women. *Breast Cancer Res Treat* 2013; 137(2): 571–7.

12. Grundy R, Larcher V, Gosden RG, et al. Fertility preservation for children treated for cancer (2): Ethics of consent for gamete storage and experimentation. *Arch Dis Child* 2001; 84: 360–2.

13. Kelleher S, Wishart SM, Liu PY, et al. Long-term outcomes of elective human sperm cryostorage. *Hum Reprod* 2001; 16: 2632–9.

14. Blackhall FH, Atkinson AD, Maaya MB, et al. Semen cryopreservation, utilisation and reproductive outcome in men treated for Hodgkin's disease. *Br J Cancer* 2002; 87(4): 381–4.

15. Donnez J, Dolmans MM, Pellicer A, et al. Restoration of ovarian activity and pregnancy after transplantation of cryopreserved ovarian tissue: A review of 60 cases of reimplantation. *Fertil Steril* 2013; 99(6): 1503–13.

16. Wallace WH, Thomson AB, Saran F, Kelsey TW. Predicting age of ovarian failure after radiation to a field that includes the ovaries. *Int J Radiat Oncol Biol Phys* 2005; 62(3): 738–44.

17. Sanders JE, Hawley J, Levy W, et al. Pregnancies following high-dose cyclophospha-mide with or without high-dose busulfan or total-body irradiation and bone marrow transplantation. *Blood* 1996; 87: 3045–52.

18. Signorello LB, Mulvihill JJ, Green DM, et al. Stillbirth and neonatal death in relation to radiation exposure before conception: A retrospective cohort study. *Lancet* 2010; 376(9741): 624–30.

19. Cobo A, Kuwayama M, Perez S, Ruiz A, Pellicer A, Remohi J. Comparison of concomitant outcome achieved with fresh and cryopreserved donor oocytes vitrified by the Cryotop method. *Fertil Steril* 2008; 89(6): 1657–64.

20. Plante M. Evolution in fertility-preserving options for early-stage cervical cancer: radical trachelectomy, simple trachelectomy, neoadjuvant chemotherapy. *Int J Gynecol Cancer* 2013; 23(6): 982–9.

21. Oktay K, Buyuk E, Davis O, Yermakova I, Veeck L, Rosenwaks Z. Fertility preservation in breast cancer patients: IVF and embryo cryopreservation after ovarian stimulation with tamoxifen. *Hum Reprod* 2003; 18: 90–5.

22. Mitwally MF, Casper RF. Aromatase inhibition reduces the dose of gonadotropin required for controlled ovarian hyperstimulation. *J Soc Gynecol Investig* 2004; 11(6): 406–15.

23. Oktay K, Hourvitz A, Sahin G, et al. Letrozole reduces estrogen and gonadotropin exposure in women with breast cancer undergoing ovarian stimulation before chemotherapy. *J Clin Endocrinol Metab* 2006; 91: 3885–90.

24. Azim AA, Costantini-Ferrando M, Oktay K. Safety of fertility preservation by ovarian stimulation with letrozole and gonadotropins in patients with breast cancer: A prospective controlled study. *J Clin Oncol* 2008; 26(16): 2630–5.

25. Azim A, Oktay K. Letrozole for ovulation induction and fertility preservation by embryo cryopreservation in young women with endometrial carcinoma. *Fertil Steril* 2007; 88(3): 657–64.

26. Anderson RA, Rosendahl M, Kelsey TW, Cameron DA. Pretreatment anti-Mullerian hormone predicts for loss of ovarian function after chemotherapy for early breast cancer. *Eur J Cancer* 2013; 49(16): 3404–11.

27. Anderson RA, Kinniburgh D, Baird DT. Preliminary evidence of the use of a gonadotrophin releasing-hormone antagonist in superovulation/IVF prior to cancer treatment. *Hum Reprod* 1999; 14: 2665–8.

28. Cakmak H, Katz A, Cedars MI, Rosen MP. Effective method for emergency fertility preservation: Random-start controlled ovarian stimulation. *Fertil Steril* 2013.

29. Nardo LG, Bosch E, Lambalk CB, Gelbaya TA. Controlled ovarian hyperstimulation regimens: a review of the available evidence for clinical practice. Produced on behalf of the BFS Policy and Practice Committee. *Hum Fertil (Camb)* 2013; 16(3): 144–50.

15

The Girl with Cancer

KT Schmidt

CONTENTS

Background

The overall survival rate after childhood cancer has improved significantly over the past decades, and thus more and more adults will be childhood cancer survivors. Subsequently, this particular group of patients will be found more frequently in fertility clinics seeking help to have a child, now and in the future. It is important to understand that women who have been treated in childhood for a cancer may present with various physical problems that can be attributed to the chemo- or radiation therapy they received as a child, and that may pose a challenge to obtaining and completing a pregnancy and delivery. Both chemotherapy and mediastinal radiation are known to cause long-term cardiac and pulmonary morbidity.[1] Cardiomyopathy and arrhythmias are well-known, albeit rare, sequelae to chemotherapy, and mediastinal radiation may cause pericardial damage. Pulmonary fibrosis is a known sequela to both radiation and chemotherapy, and all of these conditions may pose a challenge to the woman in pregnancy, where a growing foetus already makes significant demands on the mother's cardiac and pulmonary function.

Another very important point to consider is the patient's ovarian reserve. While the ovaries of young girls subjected to cancer treatment seem to be quite resistant to the gonadotoxic effects of chemotherapy and radiation therapy, girls treated for a childhood cancer are nevertheless at risk of a diminished ovarian reserve, which could negatively affect their fertility later in life. This is especially the case if they have been treated with abdominal radiation or total body irradiation or high doses of alkylating agents.[2] Because of the finite pool of primordial follicles in the ovary, formed during fetal life and exhausted at the time of menopause, a significant reduction in the number of primordial follicles due to cancer treatment in childhood may mean a risk of early menopause or premature ovarian insufficiency later in life, as this pool cannot be replenished. If all follicles in an ovary are lost, the girl will never spontaneously undergo puberty, or, if she is treated after menarche, she will become amenorrhoeic and suffer the side effects of a hypo-estrogenic milieu. Consequently, she will be sterile.

Another reproductive organ which can be affected by radiation therapy is the uterus. A pre-pubertal uterus which has been irradiated may never undergo the growth and development, which is normally seen in conjunction to oestrogenic exposure during puberty, and may as a consequence not be able to adjust to a growing foetus, with devastating obstetrical consequences such as second-trimester abortion, intra-uterine growth restriction (IUGR), premature delivery and severe haemorrhage post-partum.[3] Apart from the reduced uterine volume seen in women irradiated during childhood, myometrial fibrosis, uterine vasculature damage, and endometrial injury are common side effects to uterine irradiation directly associated to the dose given, with higher risks with increasing doses.

Impact of Condition on IVF

Ovarian Reserve

Even though they may be cycling regularly, female childhood cancer survivors are at risk of having a reduced ovarian reserve with lower ovarian volumes, lower antral follicle counts and lower anti-Müllerian hormone (AMH).[4] This means that they may experience shorter cycles, a reduced chance of obtaining a spontaneous pregnancy and, when seeking IVF, do not respond sufficiently to stimulation as is the case with low responders. Often, they require higher total doses of follicle-stimulating hormone (FSH) than age-matched fertility patients who have never received chemotherapy or radiation therapy, and a reduced response to the hormonal stimulation can be expected and thus a reduced chance of obtaining a pregnancy due to the lower numbers of obtained embryos. In Table 15.1 the consequences and risks of having received chemotherapy in childhood are listed.

Uterine Factors

A uterus which has been subjected to radiation during childhood, either as whole-abdominal, pelvic or total body irradiation, is often significantly smaller than uteri of non-irradiated patients. The volume has been found to be significantly correlated to age at treatment, with smaller volumes in those treated at younger ages.[5,6] Simultaneously, the endometrial thickness may be affected as well, but this is probably most pronounced in those who never entered puberty spontaneously due to ovarian insufficiency. In two small studies of adult childhood cancer survivors suffering from premature ovarian insufficiency (POI), who had all been subjected to whole-abdominal or pelvic irradiation, it was found that treatment for one to three months with 150 micrograms of oestradiol patches did not result in an increase in uterine size,

TABLE 15.1

Ovarian Risk of Treatment of Cancer in Childhood

Treatment	Consequence	Risk
Abdominal irradiation	Causes extensive cell damage	Failure to undergo puberty
	Follicles in an ovary highly susceptible to this damage	Premature ovarian insufficiency
		Early menopause
Cranio-spinal irradiation	Affects the hypothalamic-pituitary axis	Hypothalamic-pituitary dysfunction
		Precocious or late-onset or arrested puberty
		Growth retardation
Chemotherapy	Destroys follicles in a dose-dependent manner	Failure to undergo puberty
	Alkylating agents more gonadotoxic than other chemotherapeutic agents	Premature ovarian insufficiency
		Early menopause

TABLE 15.2

Uterine Risk of Treatment of Cancer in Childhood

Treatment	Consequence	Risk
Pre-pubertal irradiation	The uterus will not grow in size during puberty, and the muscular cells will become fibrotic.	Second-trimester abortion
		IUGR
		PROM*
		Post-partum haemorrhage
	Injured endometrium.	Unable to respond to hormones/remains thin
Post-pubertal irradiation	The uterus has undergone the normal development during puberty but may still, if the total irradiation dose is high, become fibrotic.	Second-trimester abortion
		IUGR
		PROM
		Post-partum haemorrhage
Chemotherapy	Chemotherapy does not seem to have a detrimental effect on the uterus.	None

* PROM: premature rupture of membranes.

uterine artery blood flow or endometrial thickness. Thus, it does not appear to improve pregnancy outcome to supplement with oestradiol.[5,6] Reassuringly, the endometrium in childhood cancer survivors who have a spontaneous cycle seems to respond in a normal way to the hormonal cyclical changes of the menstrual cycle. In Table 15.2 the consequences and risks of having had uterine irradiation in childhood are listed.

Impact of Condition on Pregnancy

Ovarian Factor

It does not seem that primordial follicles that survive chemotherapy or radiation therapy are damaged in any way. Thus, it is fair to assume that if a childhood cancer survivor becomes pregnant after IVF, her chances of a healthy foetus and child are the same as any other fertility patient. Since her ovarian reserve may be lower, the number of follicles that are recruited is less, and thus the chance of obtaining a healthy embryo that can implant and lead to a healthy pregnancy is reduced, but as with other young low responders it does not seem that the quality of the oocytes in these women with a low AMH is affected as much as the quantity. Reassuringly, large epidemiological studies on pregnancy outcome have shown that there is no increased risk of congenital malformations in the children of childhood cancer survivors as compared to healthy sibling controls.[7,8] There also is no increased risk of the offspring developing cancer themselves in childhood.

Uterine Factor

Preterm delivery, IUGR, second-trimester abortions and severe post-partum bleeding appear significantly more often in women who have received radiation to the uterus during childhood than in women who have only received chemotherapy or women who have never received cancer treatment. Thus, pregnancies in women with an irradiated uterus are to be considered high-risk pregnancies and should be followed closely by an obstetrical team. This risk is directly associated to age of treatment, total radiation dose and site of irradiation. The greatest risk is found in women who were very young at the time of irradiation, who had direct pelvic irradiation or total body irradiation and who received doses exceeding 14 to 30 Gy[3]. If the endometrium has been injured, it has been hypothesized that the normal decidualization may be prevented, thus leading to placental attachment disorders such as placenta accreta or percreta.

Preparing the Patient for IVF

Counselling

When counselling a childhood cancer survivor prior to IVF it is of utmost importance that she is thoroughly informed about her risks if she has received irradiation to her uterus. The risk is highest if she has received irradiation pre-pubertally. She needs to be aware that she will have a high-risk pregnancy that needs to be followed closely by an obstetrical team. Her risk of second-trimester abortion, premature delivery, premature rupture of membranes, IUGR and atonia post-partum which can result in uncontrollable post-partum haemorrhage needs to be made clear to her so that she can make her own informed choice as to whether she wants to proceed or not. If her risk is very high she may need to be discouraged of carrying a pregnancy herself, seeking other options such as adoption or a gestational carrier.

If the pelvic scan and the AMH suggest a low ovarian reserve she needs to be informed about her reduced chance of a pregnancy. If she has pulmonary or cardiac sequelae from chemotherapy or irradiation above the diaphragm, she needs to be informed if this is thought to contraindicate pregnancy.

Physical Examination

First of all, it is important to establish whether the patient still has a cycle or not. If she has been taking oral contraceptives she must stop taking these in order to properly assess her ovarian function. A pelvic ultrasound examination in order to measure the ovarian volume and number of antral follicles and to assess the uterus (size, endometrium) is recommended. Cycle day 2–5 blood tests to measure AMH, FSH

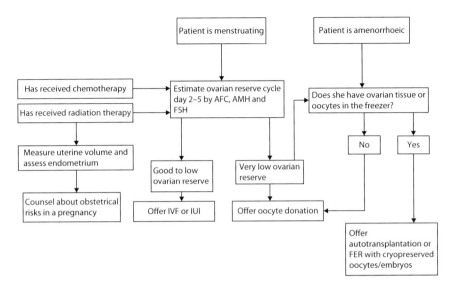

FIGURE 15.1 Considerations before offering IVF to a childhood cancer survivor.

and oestradiol are to be taken to evaluate her ovarian reserve. If the AMH is very low or the FSH is high it may be necessary to discourage her from seeking IVF as her chances of obtaining a pregnancy will be negligible. In these cases oocyte donation may be an option. In addition to tests of ovarian reserve, thyroid function should be assessed, as hypothyroidism is common in cancer survivors. Figure 15.1 is a flow chart of the considerations that should be made before offering IVF.

Fertility Preservation

Although fertility preservation in girls is difficult and is often not performed, there are ways to preserve the fertility even in young patients.[9] Ovarian tissue cryopreservation is the only valid way to preserve fertility in pre-pubertal girls. Although no children have yet been born to women who had their ovarian tissue cryopreserved in childhood, there are encouraging results from autotransplantation of cryopreserved ovarian tissue in adult women both in terms of restoration of ovarian function and in the delivery of babies. In the sexually active post-pubertal girl cryopreservation of embryos (fertilized with donor sperm) or vitrification of oocytes may be an option. Increasing numbers of childhood cancer survivors, who have previously undergone some sort of fertility preservation prior to oncological treatment, are now presenting for fertility treatment and requesting the use of their cryopreserved oocytes or embryos in order to become pregnant. However, as yet only a few, very small studies reporting the outcome of IVF in cancer patients who have had oocytes or embryos cryopreserved have been published. If cryopreserved ovarian tissue is available the patient should be referred to a centre with the expertise to autotransplant this tissue, which would typically be the centre in which the actual cryopreservation took place. If she has embryos or oocytes in the freezer these can be used in a frozen embryo replacement cycle to obtain a pregnancy.

Management in Early Pregnancy

If the patient is already under the care of a long-term oncology follow-up clinic it is important to let them know that she is pregnant so that she can be followed there with more frequent controls if necessary. A high-risk pregnancy should always be referred early to a specialised obstetrical team. This is especially the case in women with an irradiated uterus. If there are additional medical problems such as hypothyroidism, the patient should be referred to an endocrinologist or a specialist in internal medicine. In most cases however, a woman who has received chemotherapy for a cancer in childhood can be reassured that she is likely to experience an uneventful pregnancy and deliver a healthy baby.

REFERENCES

1. Mertens AC, Yasui Y, Neglia JP, et al. Late mortality experience in five-year survivors of childhood and adolescent cancer: The Childhood Cancer Survivor Study. *J Clin Oncol* 2001;19:3163–72.
2. Sklar CA, Mertens AC, Mitby P, et al. Premature menopause in survivors of childhood cancer: A report from the Childhood Cancer Survivor Study. *J Natl Cancer Inst* 2006;98:890–6.
3. Wo JY, Viswanathan AN. Impact of radiotherapy on fertility, pregnancy, and neonatal outcomes in female cancer patients. *Int J Radiat Oncol Biol Phys* 2009;73:1304–12.
4. Nielsen SN, Andersen AN, Schmidt KT, et al. A 10-year follow up of reproductive function in women treated for childhood cancer. *RBMonline* 2013;27:192–200.
5. Larsen EC, Schmiegelow K, Rechnitzer C, et al. Radiotherapy at a young age reduces uterine volume of childhood cancer survivors. *Acta Obstet Gynecol Scand* 2004;83:96–102.
6. Critchley HOD, Wallace WHB, Shalet SM, et al. Abdominal irradiation in childhood; the potential for pregnancy. *Br J Obstet Gynaecol* 1992;99:392–4.
7. Green DM, Sklar CA, Boice JD Jr, et al. Ovarian failure and reproductive outcomes after childhood cancer treatment: Results from the Childhood Cancer Survivor Study. *J Clin Oncol* 2009;27:2374–81.
8. Mulvihill JJ, Connelly RR, Austin DF, et al. Cancer in offspring of long-term survivors of childhood and adolescent cancer. *Lancet* 1987;2:813–7.
9. Schmidt KT, Larsen EC, Andersen CY, et al. Risk of ovarian failure and fertility preserving methods in girls and adolescents with a malignant disease. *BJOG* 2010;117:163–74.

16

The Patient with Turner's Syndrome

O Hovatta and B Borgström

CONTENTS

Background

A characteristic feature in Turner's syndrome is ovarian failure.[1] Girls with Turner's syndrome have normal numbers of primordial follicles in their ovaries up to the middle of the fetal period. These numbers then start to diminish, but some 40% of Turner women have at least some oocytes remaining as they enter early childhood and the teenage years.[2–4] Positive predictors for having residual ovarian follicles at puberty are a mosaic karyotype, spontaneous onset of puberty, and normal serum concentration of follicle-stimulating hormone (FSH) and anti-Mullerian hormone (AMH).[1]

Recent reports[1,5,6] indicated that around 12% of women with Turner's syndrome conceive ongoing pregnancies, and spontaneous conceptions appear to be as frequently encountered as those achieved by oocyte donation. Interestingly, half of a cohort of 115 Swedish women with Turner's syndrome who had children had not been diagnosed as having the syndrome before the pregnancy. In a Danish study based on a cytogenetics registry (1973–1993), of 410 Turner women, 31 (7.6%) had achieved a spontaneous pregnancy.[7]

However, the majority of women with Turner's syndrome presenting to the reproductive endocrinologist expressing a desire to conceive will require *in vitro* fertilization with donated oocytes.

Impact of Turner's Syndrome on IVF

When girls with Turner's syndrome have achieved spontaneous menarche, it is possible to collect mature oocytes and cryostore them by vitrification. This necessitates ovarian stimulation with exogenous gonadotropins and a transvaginal oocyte retrieval procedure. Any oocytes obtained can then be vitrified for thaw and fertilization when the woman decides she wishes to conceive.[12,13] However, many of these patients do not have many follicles remaining after menarche, making ovarian stimulation of sufficient follicles to provide a reasonable chance of pregnancy via in vitro fertilization (IVF) difficult. The risk of ovarian hyperstimulation syndrome (OHSS) is not high even though the girls/women may be of small size.

In the case of ovarian failure, excellent pregnancy rates can be achieved using oocyte donation.[1,9]

Impact of IVF and Pregnancy on Turner's Syndrome

There are a number of safety concerns regarding pregnancies in Turner women. A key concern relates to the haemodynamic changes during pregnancy, which may increase the risk of aortic dilation and rupture. However, since these life-threatening events occur commonly in Turner women who are not pregnant, it is unclear to what extent pregnancy increases the risk of these serious aortal events. While recent North European and North American data have been reassuring[6,20] further large-registry-based information is needed.

Turner's syndrome is associated with a number of cardiac anomalies, including bicuspid aortic valve and aortic coarctation.[14-16] These women often have high blood pressure and are prone to aortic dilation and dissection[17,18] which can be fatal. This complication is a commonly reported cause of early death among women with Turner's syndrome.[6,19-21] While it can occur without pregnancy, a number of case reports highlighted the risk of it happening during pregnancy or close to pregnancy.[18,22-24]

When pregnancies are induced by IVF, the risk of complications can be reduced by carrying out single-embryo transfer. Advances in cryopreservation techniques render this a feasible approach which need not reduce the chance of the woman conceiving. In addition to reducing the haemodynamic challenge of pregnancy compared with that imposed by multiples, singleton pregnancies are advisable to avoid the mechanical burdens that multiple pregnancy can bring to women with Turner's, who often have a small stature.

Preparing the Patient for IVF

Careful medical health control is compulsory before a pregnancy in Turner's syndrome, irrespective of whether it is a planned spontaneous pregnancy or IVF using the patient's own or donated oocytes. Women with Turner's syndrome may present with a number of concurrent medical conditions (Table 16.1) which require assessment and management prior to starting treatment. Preconceptional

TABLE 16.1

Medical Problems Associated with Turner's Syndrome

Cardiovascular disease (40%)
Bicuspid aortic valve
Aortic coarctation
Aortic dilatation 8–28%
Hypertension (40%)
Hyperlipidaemia (50%)
Insulin resistance: type 2 diabetes twice as common
Hypothyroidism (25%)
Renal disorders (30% structural anomaly)

TABLE 16.2

Pre-pregnancy Screening in Turner's Syndrome

Cardiovascular examination (including echocardiogram and magnetic resonance imaging)
Glucose challenge test
Liver and thyroid function tests
Screening for autoimmune disorders (Hashimoto's thyroidism and Addison's disease)

expert cardiovascular assessment is mandatory. Complications can be avoided by proper follow-up and by abstaining from pregnancy if the risk of aortic rupture is regarded as high.[22] The risk of the most severe complication, aortic rupture, has to be evaluated before and during pregnancy by measuring the aortic root using magnetic resonance imaging (MRI), also during pregnancy. It is also important to check thyroid function, blood sugar status and liver function prior to commencing treatment (Table 16.2).

Management during IVF Treatment

For those undergoing IVF either to conceive with their own oocytes or to cryostore oocytes for later use, ovarian stimulation regimens should be individualized, taking into account the antral follicle count, serum AMH level, FSH concentrations, and the size of the woman. Transvaginal oocyte retrieval can be performed according to normal procedure, but blood pressure should be monitored through treatment. The majority of women with Turner's syndrome will however need donor oocytes to conceive. To ensure adequate uterine maturation, cyclic estrogen-progesterone treatment should be offered for some six months before the planned treatment to Turner's patients who do not have regular spontaneous cycles.

Management in Pregnancy

These are high-risk pregnancies, and they require continuous close follow-up. Regular blood pressure and blood sugar and thyroid hormone measurements are even more important than among other pregnant women. The aortic root also requires frequent measurement during pregnancy, and it is recommended that this be checked by MRI or ultrasound each trimester. If there is progressive dilation, operative intervention to end the pregnancy should be considered.

In spite of the existing risks, North European pregnancy results have been reassuring, with only one aortic rupture during pregnancy among hundreds of known cases. Fortunately that case resulted in healthy mother and baby.

The well-known risks in the pregnancies of women with Turner's syndrome have to be taken into account when a woman with Turner's syndrome is planning a pregnancy, during pregnancy and after the pregnancy. Complications can be avoided by proper follow-up.[22]

The incidence of miscarriages in both spontaneous[5,8] and oocyte donation-derived pregnancies[9] has been high. However, adequate hormonal replacement therapy (HRT) given to these women to allow the uterus to mature prior to attempting oocyte donation can reduce this risk.

Other Options for Conception

In addition to oocyte donation, other options aimed at helping girls and women with Turner's syndrome to become pregnant are now emerging. One approach in which experience is growing is the cryopreservation of ovarian cortical tissue and transplantation of the tissue back to the ovary at the time pregnancy is desired. Recent studies indicated that there is little value in performing ovarian tissue removal and cryopreservation very early in life. The optimal age for cryopreservation of the tissue appears to be 12–14 years,[2,5] as younger girls have not been found to have significantly large amounts of eggs in the ovarian cortex. In our experience, it is usually possible to isolate immature oocytes from the biopsied tissue and freeze them separately, but as yet we have not proceeded to fertilize such immature eggs. Cryopreservation of aspirated oocytes matured *in vitro* from a Turner's patient has been reported,[10] but the data remain preliminary.

When the Turner woman desires children, the frozen tissue can in principle be transplanted to her ovary or some other site. This procedure has been developed and extensively applied and reported in women as a means of preserving fertility prior to undergoing gonadotoxic anti-cancer treatments. Ovarian cryopreservation and transplantation in this context has so far resulted in some 30 reported pregnancies with children born among women without Turner's. Experience in Turner's syndrome is at present far less. We have transplanted biopsied frozen-thawed tissue to one Turner woman who unfortunately had very few follicles in the tissue. No return of ovarian function was achieved. However, another group has reported a live birth after transplantation of ovarian cortical tissue from a discordant twin sister to a sister who had Turner's syndrome.[11] If no oocytes can be obtained from ovarian biopsy material and the woman has undergone early ovarian failure, it is still possible to help her to become pregnant by using donated oocytes. The pregnancy rates after egg donation are similar among women with Turner syndrome as those reported in women with other causes of ovarian failure.

Almost all women with Turner's syndrome suffer from premature ovarian failure. Hence these women should be counselled not to unnecessarily postpone childbearing. The following short case history is illustrative of this point.

Case History

A girl with Turner's syndrome was referred to our fertility unit at the age of 12 years by a paediatric endocrinologist. She participated in a study designed to discern which girls might benefit from ovarian tissue freezing for fertility preservation. In this study, putative prognostic factors such as age, AMH levels and karyotype were tested for their ability to predict the number of follicles found in ovarian tissue obtained from the same subjects.[2] The girl was found to have ovarian follicles in the cortical tissue. Most of the biopsied tissue was frozen for fertility preservation.

This girl was considered to have a relatively good prognosis for ovarian function because follicles were found. Her karyotype was 45, X, but only 10 metaphase cells had been analyzed. It is possible that she had a mosaic Turner's syndrome. She received careful counselling regarding the possibilities of having pregnancies and children. This included a recommendation not to unnecessarily postpone childbearing. She went into spontaneous menarche at the age of 14.

While still in her teens, she entered a relationship with a boy of the same age. These two young individuals had families who supported their expressed desire to have children, and she conceived spontaneously at the age of 18. The pregnancy was carefully followed up, and she had a prenatal chromosome test from amniotic fluid. MRI and ultrasound scan did not reveal any signs of aortic dilation. Her blood pressure remained normal, as did her blood glucose levels and thyroid function. She delivered a healthy baby boy with a normal weight at term.

At the age of 20, this young mother conceived again and delivered a baby girl. Her health remained good, with normal blood pressure and endocrine health. However, at the age of 22 years she underwent premature ovarian failure and was treated with estrogen-progesterone replacement. Annual health controls were instigated. The frozen-stored ovarian tissue remains in cryostorage in a gas-phase liquid nitrogen tank.

Key Practice Points

1. Some 40% of Turner's syndrome teenagers still have eggs in their ovaries.
2. Positive prognostic signs for having eggs are the beginning of spontaneous pubertal development, mosaic Turner's syndrome, and normal serum concentrations of FSH and AMH, but none of them is exclusive.
3. Pregnancies have been encountered among Turner women who never had menarche. The girl should be informed about this, and oral contraceptives should be considered as HRT if she opts for that.
4. Turner women undergo early ovarian failure and they should be informed not to unnecessarily postpone childbearing.
5. IVF is feasible for women with Turner's syndrome who still have ovarian function.
6. Egg donation is an effective method to treat the infertility of Turner women who already have undergone ovarian failure.

7. Turner's syndrome women have a high risk of aortic dilation and rupture, particularly if they have bicuspid aortic valve and/or aortic coarctation. It is not known if a pregnancy increases this risk, but the hemodynamic changes during pregnancy may be a risk factor.

8. Only one embryo at a time should be transferred because of the greater associated hemodynamic changes in multiple pregnancies.

9. Preconceptional expert cardiovascular assessment is mandatory. The risk of aortic rupture has to be evaluated before and during pregnancy by measuring the aortic root using MRI, also during pregnancy.

10. When considering fertility preservation by ovarian tissue cryopreservation, this should be done at around 12–14 years of age.

REFERENCES

1. Hovatta O. Ovarian function and *in vitro* fertilization (IVF) in Turner syndrome. *Pediatric Endocrinology Reviews*: PER. 2012 May;9 Suppl 2:713–7. PubMed PMID: 22946282.

2. Borgstrom B, Hreinsson J, Rasmussen C, Sheikhi M, Fried G, Keros V, et al. Fertility preservation in girls with Turner syndrome: Prognostic signs of the presence of ovarian follicles. *Journal of Clinical Endocrinology and Metabolism*. 2009 Jan;94(1):74–80. PubMed PMID: 18957497.

3. Hagman A, Wennerholm UB, Kallen K, Barrenas ML, Landin-Wilhelmsen K, Hanson C, et al. Women who gave birth to girls with Turner syndrome: Maternal and neonatal characteristics. *Human Reproduction*. 2010 Jun;25(6):1553–60. PubMed PMID: 20237051.

4. Hreinsson JG, Otala M, Fridstrom M, Borgstrom B, Rasmussen C, Lundqvist M, et al. Follicles are found in the ovaries of adolescent girls with Turner's syndrome. *Journal of Clinical Endocrinology and Metabolism*. 2002 Aug;87(8):3618–23. PubMed PMID: 12161485.

5. Bryman I, Sylven L, Berntorp K, Innala E, Bergstrom I, Hanson C, et al. Pregnancy rate and outcome in Swedish women with Turner syndrome. *Fertility and Sterility*. 2011 Jun 30;95(8):2507–10. PubMed PMID: 21256486.

6. Hadnott TN, Gould HN, Gharib AM, Bondy CA. Outcomes of spontaneous and assisted pregnancies in Turner syndrome: The U.S. National Institutes of Health experience. *Fertility and Sterility*. 2011 Jun;95(7):2251–6. PubMed PMID: 21496813. Pubmed Central PMCID: 3130000.

7. Birkebaek NH, Cruger D, Hansen J, Nielsen J, Bruun-Petersen G. Fertility and pregnancy outcome in Danish women with Turner syndrome. *Clinical Genetics*. 2002 Jan;61(1):35–9. PubMed PMID: 11903353.

8. Hovatta O. Pregnancies in women with Turner's syndrome. *Annals of Medicine*. 1999 Apr;31(2):106–10. PubMed PMID: 10344582.

9. Foudila T, Soderstrom-Anttila V, Hovatta O. Turner's syndrome and pregnancies after oocyte donation. *Human Reproduction*. 1999 Feb;14(2):532–5. PubMed PMID: 10100005.

10. Lau NM, Huang JY, MacDonald S, Elizur S, Gidoni Y, Holzer H, et al. Feasibility of fertility preservation in young females with Turner syndrome. *Reproductive Biomedicine Online*. 2009 Feb;18(2):290–5. PubMed PMID: 19192353.

11. Donnez J, Dolmans MM, Squifflet J, Kerbrat G, Jadoul P. Live birth after allografting of ovarian cortex between monozygotic twins with Turner syndrome

(45,XO/46,XX mosaicism) and discordant ovarian function. *Fertility and Sterility.* 2011 Dec;96(6):1407–11. PubMed PMID: 21982291.

12. Oktay K, Rodriguez-Wallberg KA, Sahin G. Fertility preservation by ovarian stimulation and oocyte cryopreservation in a 14-year-old adolescent with Turner syndrome mosaicism and impending premature ovarian failure. *Fertility and Sterility.* 2010 Jul;94(2):753 e15–9. PubMed PMID: 20188362.

13. El-Shawarby SA, Sharif F, Conway G, Serhal P, Davies M. Oocyte cryopreservation after controlled ovarian hyperstimulation in mosaic Turner syndrome: Another fertility preservation option in a dedicated UK clinic. *BJOG: An International Journal of Obstetrics and Gynaecology.* 2010 Jan;117(2):234–7. PubMed PMID: 20002398.

14. Lippe B. Turner syndrome. *Endocrinology and Metabolism Clinics of North America.* 1991 Mar;20(1):121–52. PubMed PMID: 2029883.

15. Lopez L, Arheart KL, Colan SD, Stein NS, Lopez-Mitnik G, Lin AE, et al. Turner syndrome is an independent risk factor for aortic dilation in the young. *Pediatrics.* 2008 Jun;121(6):E1622–E7. PubMed PMID: WOS:000256313700023. English.

16. Mortensen KH, Erlandsen M, Andersen NH, Gravholt CH. Prediction of aortic dilation in Turner syndrome – enhancing the use of serial cardiovascular magnetic resonance. *Journal of Cardiovascular Magnetic Resonance: Official Journal of the Society for Cardiovascular Magnetic Resonance.* 2013 Jun 6;15(1):47. PubMed PMID: 23742092. Pubmed Central PMCID: 3702474.

17. Birdsall M, Kennedy S. The risk of aortic dissection in women with Turner syndrome. *Human Reproduction.* 1996 Jul;11(7):1587. PubMed PMID: 8671511.

18. Gravholt CH, Landin-Wilhelmsen K, Stochholm K, Hjerrild BE, Ledet T, Djurhuus CB, et al. Clinical and epidemiological description of aortic dissection in Turner's syndrome. *Cardiology in the Young.* 2006 Oct;16(5):430–6. PubMed PMID: 16984695.

19. Carlson M, Airhart N, Lopez L, Silberbach M. Moderate aortic enlargement and bicuspid aortic valve are associated with aortic dissection in Turner syndrome: Report of the International Turner Syndrome Aortic Dissection Registry. *Circulation.* 2012 Oct 30;126(18):2220–6. PubMed PMID: 23032325.

20. Hagman A, Kallen K, Bryman I, Landin-Wilhelmsen K, Barrenas ML, Wennerholm UB. Morbidity and mortality after childbirth in women with Turner karyotype. *Human Reproduction.* 2013 Jul;28(7):1961–73. PubMed PMID: 23578947.

21. Karnis MF. Catastrophic consequences of assisted reproduction: The case of Turner syndrome. *Seminars in Reproductive Medicine.* 2012 Apr;30(2):116–22. PubMed PMID: 22549711.

22. Bondy CA, Turner Syndrome Study Group. Care of girls and women with Turner syndrome: A guideline of the Turner Syndrome Study Group. *Journal of Clinical Endocrinology and Metabolism.* 2007 Jan;92(1):10–25. PubMed PMID: 17047017.

23. Chevalier N, Bstandig B, Galand-Portier M, Isnard V, Bongain A, Fenichel P. [Oocyte donation in patients with Turner syndrome: A high-risk pregnancy]. *Annales d'Endocrinologie.* 2009 Sep;70(4):246–51. PubMed PMID: 19200942. Procreation par don d'ovocytes dans le syndrome de Turner: Une situation a haut risque.

24. Landin-Wilhelmsen K, Bryman I, Hanson C, Hanson L. Spontaneous pregnancies in a Turner syndrome woman with Y-chromosome mosaicism. *Journal of Assisted Reproduction and Genetics.* 2004 Jun;21(6):229–30. PubMed PMID: 15526979. Pubmed Central PMCID: 3455230.

17

The Couple Testing Positive for Hepatitis B and C

JG Lemmen, A Loft, and S Ziebe

CONTENTS

Background

With the implementation of the EU cell and tissue directive from 2006 into national legislation it became mandatory to screen all fertility patients for HIV and hepatitis B virus (HBV) (hepatitis B surface antigen [HBsAg] and total hepatitis B core antibody [anti-HBc]) and hepatitis C virus (HCV) (hepatitis C virus antibody [anti-HCV]) prior to initiating fertility treatment. However, it was stated in the directive that "positive results will not necessarily prevent partner donation in accordance with national rules". As a consequence of this, fertility clinics all over Europe are now contacted by viral-positive patients seeking help to conceive by assisted reproduction technology (ART).

However, treatment with ART in couples where one or both partners are hepatitis positive raises concern about transfer of the infection to others (i.e. a partner, the baby, the other patients or the staff at the fertility clinic).

Generally, the risk of transferring a virus to other couples during treatment with assisted reproduction is considered extremely low (Wingfield and Cottell 2010). It is however still important to identify unacknowledged infected couples to ensure counselling and proper neonatal care to prevent vertical transmission of the virus to the child.

In this chapter we focus on the practical aspects of treating viral-positive patients, and consequently this is not a comprehensive review of what is a very complex area of medicine.

It is therefore essential to underline the importance of close collaboration with experts in viral infections when offering ART to viral-positive patients.

Prevalence and Transmission of the Virus

Hepatitis B

HBV is a double-stranded DNA virus with a prevalence of approximately 2% in Western Europe. Areas with a high prevalence (more than 8%) include Southeast Asia and the Pacific Basin (excluding Japan, Australia, and New Zealand), sub-Saharan Africa, the Amazon Basin, parts of the Middle East, the central Asian republics, and some countries in Eastern Europe.

HBV replicates primarily in hepatocytes, interferes with hepatic function, and also affects cells in the bone marrow. HBV-DNA can integrate into the genome of the host cell. The virus is primarily transmitted by blood, sexual activity (horizontal transmission) and during labour from mother to child, with about 5% being infected prior to delivery (vertical transmission). The incubation time is 6 to 24 weeks. The risk of developing a chronic HBV infection depends on age at time of infection; a perinatal infection carries a risk of up to 90% (depending on the viral load in the mother's blood), while less than 10% of adults develop chronicity. A subclinical infection is associated with a higher risk of developing chronicity than an acute infection. Immune-incompetence and co-infection with HIV or HCV are other risk factors for chronicity.

If a person is proven HBsAg positive for more than 6 months, she/he is classified as a chronic carrier. Chronic HBV may progress to liver fibrosis, cirrhosis and hepatocellular carcinoma. The progression of the liver disease is associated with the level of virus replication (HBV-DNA) in the blood.

Hepatitis C

HCV is an RNA virus and is found worldwide, with some countries having chronic infection rates as high as 5% and more. Prevalence in Western Europe is approximately 2%.

HCV replication occurs primarily in the liver cells. The main mode of transmission is attributed to unsafe injections using contaminated equipment or non-screened blood or blood products. Sexual transmission is low (estimated as 2.5%/10 years), and in a steady relationship the use of a condom in connection with vaginal intercourse is generally not warranted. In case of several partners, genital lesion, anal intercourse or intercourse during menstruation it is advised to use a condom. The incubation time ranges from 4 weeks to 12 weeks. About 50–80% of the cases with acute HCV develop into chronicity. Chronic HCV may progress to liver fibrosis, cirrhosis and hepatocellular carcinoma. Risk factors for cirrhosis are co-infection, age, gender (male) and alcohol intake.

Vertical transmission of HCV occurs in around 5% of pregnancies and seems to be dependent on HCV-RNA status of the mother. Chronic HCV infection is defined as the presence of HCV-RNA in the blood for more than 6 months.

Viral Testing

Patients identified to be hepatitis positive who have been seen by specialists in infectious disease management and who are considered stable can reasonably be treated in the fertility clinic.

However, as a consequence of implementation of mandatory screening of infertile patients for HBV and HCV, detection of infected and potentially contagious patients occurs. A positive test in this context should always result in referral of the patient to an infectious disease department for specific guidance regarding prognosis and potential medical treatment for their viral disease before initiating fertility treatment. Donation of gametes to other persons than their partner is generally not recommended.

Interpreting Hepatitis Screening Results

Hepatitis B Virus

Correct interpretation of the screening results is the key to counselling the patient.

If one of the screening tests (HBsAg or total anti-HBc) is positive, further investigations and referral to an infectious disease department are indicated to identify the phase of the disease.

An overview of the various scenarios which can be encountered on extended testing following positive screening is provided in Table 17.1, which also indicates the infectivity status associated with each combination of results.

HBV-DNA is a marker of active viral replication, determining infectivity of HBV carriers. As a well-recognized clinical phenomenon, persistent detectable viral genome (HBV-DNA) in liver or sera in the absence of other serological markers for active hepatitis B virus replication is termed *occult HBV infection*. The main mechanism through which occult infection occurs is not completely understood, and several possible explanations, such as integration into the genome and maintenance in peripheral mononuclear cells, exist. In a recent publication, almost 5% of HBV-vaccinated infants born to HBsAg-positive mothers were reported to acquire an occult HBV infection, with 1.6% becoming HBs-Ag positive despite the vaccination (Su et al. 2013).

TABLE 17.1

Interpretation of Hepatitis Antigen and Antibody Test Results

| | Antigens | | Antibodies | | | | | Infectious (Yes/No) |
| | HBsAg | HBeAg | Anti-HBc | | | Anti-HBs | Anti-HBe | |
			Total	IgM	IgG			
Never exposed	−	−	−	−	−	−	−	No
Incubation phase	+	+/−	−	−	−	−	−	Yes
Acute infection	+	+	+	+	−	−	−	Yes
Acute infection ("HBe window")	+	−	+	+	−	−	−	Yes
Acute infection ("core only" window)	−	−	+	+	−	−	+	Yes
Resolved HBV infection	−	−	+	−	+	+	+	No
Chronic HBV	+	+	+	−	+	−	−	Yes
Chronic HBV	+	−	+	−	+	−	+	Yes
Previous HBV	−	−	+	−	+	−	−	?
Occult HBV	−	−	+	−	+	−	−	?
False positive	−	−	+	−	+	−	−	No
HBV vaccinated	−	−	−	−	−	+	−	No

Note: HBeAg, hepatitis Be antigen: marker of an active infection (acute or chronic), determining infectivity of HBV carriers, can pass through the placenta before labour and lead to chronic hepatitis after delivery despite vaccination and immunoglobulin.

Anti-HBc IgM, IgM antibody against the core (nucleus) of the hepatitis B virus.

Anti-HBc IgC, IgC antibody against the core (nucleus) of the hepatitis B virus.

Anti-HBs, hepatitis B surface antibody: antibody against the surface of the hepatitis B virus. As vaccination against hepatitis B is only carried out with an empty "shell" of virus, people who are vaccinated only make anti-HBs antibodies.

Anti-HBe, hepatitis Be antibody: marker of previous infection or late phase of chronic infection.

Hepatitis C Virus

If the patient has antibodies against HCV (anti-HCV), a polymerase chain reaction (PCR) technique is used to confirm positivity and to diagnose active replication (HCV-RNA). If replication is proven then the patient is regarded as infectious. In the inactive stage of the disease, patients are found to be HCV antibody positive with normal liver function but PCR negative. The presence of HCV antibodies does not protect against a re-infection with HCV.

Vaccination

Hepatitis B Virus

An effective vaccination programme is available for HBV. In couples in whom only one of the partners is HBV positive it is advised that the negative partner has completed the vaccination programme (day 0, 1 and 6 month) before onset of fertility treatment. When a child is born to an HBV-infected mother, a vaccination programme for the child (on day 0, 1, 2 and 12 months) together with an injection of HBV immunoglobulin should start immediately and not later than 48 hours after labour.

All in vitro fertilisation (IVF) unit staff should be vaccinated against HBV. After HBV vaccination the far majority (95%) will develop antibodies against the virus (anti-HBs). Medical treatment for HBV prior to onset of fertility treatment is generally not considered necessary but may be indicated after consultation with an infectious disease specialist.

Hepatitis C Virus

At present no vaccination programme against HCV is available. However, it has been suggested that if either partner is chronically infected with HCV (HCV-RNA positive), treatment with peg-interferon alpha and ribavirin should be considered and finalized *prior* to initiating assisted reproduction in order to reduce the infected partner's viral load (Foster 2004).

Impact of Disease on IVF and Pregnancy

Female fertility is not significantly affected by HBV infection unless the patient has suffered from liver failure (Piratvisuth 2013). Consequently, couples referred for fertility treatment who have unsuccessfully tried to conceive at home should be regarded as subfertile due to standard causes, rather than secondary to their hepatitis status. If the partner has been successfully vaccinated, carriers of HBV do not require barrier contraception to prevent transmission.

Usually, chronic HBV infection does not worsen during pregnancy. However cholestasis, chronic HBV flares with or without HBeAg (hepatitis Be-antigen) seroconversion and liver failure have been described during pregnancy and the peripartum period. The effect of chronic HBV infection on pregnancy outcome is not clear. A large study showed no effects on prematurity, birth weight, perinatal mortality, neonatal jaundice or anomalies (Wong et al. 1999). However, a higher risk of diabetes and antepartum haemorrhage and threatened preterm delivery have been described in women testing positive for HBsAg (Tse et al. 2005). Pregnant women with cirrhosis have an increased risk of spontaneous abortion and perinatal complications such as gestational hypertension, placental abruption and peripartum haemorrhage.

Little data is available in regard to the impact of HBV infection on the chance of successfully conceiving after fertility treatment. Some studies have demonstrated reduced sperm motility and poorer sperm morphology in HBV-positive males undergoing IVF compared to other couples undergoing IVF treatment (Lee et al. 2010, Oger et al. 2011, Zhou et al. 2011). Generally however, there is no reported impact of HBV infection on hormonal response or pregnancy success with ART (Lee et al. 2010, Chen et al. 2013). Indeed Lam et al. (2010) showed a surprisingly higher pregnancy rate for couples positive for hepatitis B.

Regarding HCV, a recent study suggested a negative impact of HCV infection (especially PCR-positive cases) on ovarian response and pregnancy rate (Hanafi et al. 2011), and an older study also showed a negative impact of HCV on IVF outcome (Englert et al. 2007). Active HCV replication may have an impact on estrogen levels and progesterone metabolism. In the case of HCV-positive males normal fertility has been reported.

Impact of IVF and Pregnancy on Disease

In general women testing positive for HBV have no increased incidence of complications during pregnancy (Jonas 2009). One study has reported no significant differences in HBV viraemia during pregnancy (Söderström et al. 2003). Pregnancy itself may have a positive effect on the HCV infection of the woman, with decreased hepatocyte damage possibly due to increased estrogen levels. Few data are available describing the impact of IVF treatment on the progress of HBV and HCV.

Preparing the Patient for IVF

Investigations and treatment for IVF should be carried out according to standard guidelines for subfertile couples.

Stimulation

Female Hepatitis Patients

Hormonal stimulation can be done in the same way as for other patients if female hepatitis patients have normal liver function. If the patient's liver function is affected, cautious ovarian stimulation is needed to avoid the risk of ovarian hyperstimulation syndrome. Clomiphene stimulation is contraindicated. After vaginal scanning, the scanner should be cleaned according to national/local hygiene guidelines. At Rigshospitalet, Copenhagen, the current recommendations are that the scanner is cleaned with a paper serviette, then a soap-containing antiseptic serviette and finally 70% alcohol.

Management during IVF Treatment

The risk of transmission of viruses during IVF is normally considered extremely low. Consequently, recommendations are often based on theoretical risk assessments rather than being evidence based. In recent years recommendations regarding safe practice have loosened compared with those previously advised. The result may therefore be that safety precautions once considered justified are considered disproportionate for today's standards.

However, gaining the confidence to change an established system is a long process. The approach to management presented in this chapter is based on current practice at Rigshospitalet, Copenhagen.

As a consequence of lack of solid data on actual risks, our current practice is based more on a safety-first principle and historical practice rather than on an actual risk assessment.

We suggest that patient records, stimulation schemes and laboratory schemes are designed in a way which makes it readily identifiable whether an individual patient or couple should be treated according to the protocol for infectious patients. At Rigshospitalet we use a colour-coding system.

Female Hepatitis Patients

At Rigshospitalet, our protocol has been developed in close collaboration with the hospital unit for hygiene. The operating room is located adjacent to our special laboratory unit for infectious patients with a small window in the wall through which follicular fluid (or embryos at transfer) are passed. The oocyte pickup is carried out according to routine protocol, but a large piece of absorbent material is placed at the floor under the patient, together with a trash container, so that in case of blood spilling, everything is absorbed. When a blood spill does occur, cleaning is performed in the same way as for the ultrasound scanner, as described previously. The doctor, nurses and lab technicians use white coats of paper/plastic, face mask, glasses and gloves which together with all-paper draping are handled as contaminated and disposed as such. The ultrasound guidance set is rinsed with hydrogen peroxide and machine washed immediately after use.

The follicular fluid may be handled in the laboratory as for other patients; however in our special unit for infectious patients we use a class II laminar flow bench. Prick injuries with contaminated material are the main cause for occupational infection with hepatitis (Gerberding and Hendersson 1992). Therefore, glassware should be avoided for all laboratory procedures to prevent infection by prick injury. Use instead plastic pipettes for handling of semen, follicular fluid and embryos. The only place where glass cannot be avoided is the ICSI (intracytoplasmic sperm injection) micropipettes. Denudation of oocyte-cumulus complexes should be carried out using plastic disposable pipettes.

Male Hepatitis Patients

For semen preparation it is advised to do a double purification procedure consisting of a gradient centrifuge step with sperm washes followed by a "swim-up" purification.

This will reduce the viral load in the semen samples to undetectable or almost undetectable, and the sample can then be handled with the same level of care as for all other biologic material. In our practice the semen sample is not tested for viral load after purification since the partner of HBV-positive males will have been vaccinated prior to treatment, and HCV couples in a steady relationship will already have been exposed to transmission risk by intercourse.

In some countries it is advised not to perform ICSI in couples where the male is HBV positive due to a possible integration of the HBV in the embryonic genome after ICSI. However, HBV in oocytes and embryos has been reported after IVF as well as ICSI, suggesting the possibility of vertical HBV transmission via both male and female infected germ cells (Nie et al. 2011, Hu et al. 2011). Again, even after natural conception it is possible that viral DNA will integrate (Tajiri et al. 2007), so there seems to be no reason to specifically advise against ICSI in chronic HBV carriers (Lutgens et al. 2009, Nie et al. 2011).

For an HCV-positive male again there is no clear contra-indication against ICSI treatment as it is known that even in natural conception integration of HCV in the embryonic genome may occur and no increase after ICSI is expected (NVOG guidelines 2010). There are no data to suggest a possible higher frequency of transmission of virus with IVF/ICSI techniques as compared to natural conception. In a large French study it has been shown that even though 20% of semen samples contained HCV-RNA, after double purification no HCV-RNA could be detected in the final sperm fraction (Bourlet et al. 2009). Moreover, none of the children born in this study were infected with HCV.

Some authors do not consider HCV to be sexually transmitted and therefore do not advise double purification. However, most publications describe the use of double purification of semen in HCV-discordant couples. The majority do not perform a nested PCR to detect HCV-RNA.

In our setup, oocyte and embryo culture are done in incubators separate from those used in non-infected patients. This precaution is not because of any risk of transmission of virus between samples located in the same incubator, but rather as a precaution of any theoretical consequence in the unlikely and rare event of mixing up embryos. Gilling-Smith and colleagues (2005) proposed that it seems "safer and more ethically acceptable to handle patients with the same level of risk together, ... , rather than mix patients with clearly different risk levels". The fact that HBV has been detected in human embryos would appear to further support this approach (Nie et al. 2011, Hu et al. 2011).

Cryopreservation

At the time of writing, there have not been any documented cases of HBV or HCV transmission during cryostorage in human IVF, so this remains a theoretical risk at this time. In a recent study by Cobo et al. (2012) no traces of virus were detectable in either spent culture medium after culture of embryos from viral-positive patients or in the liquid nitrogen after cryostorage of embryos from viral-positive patients. In our clinic, cryopreservation of surplus embryos is done in separate tanks for cryostorage intended for infectious patients; another option is with sealed straws in the same tank. To completely avoid the potential risk of contamination there is also the option of not offering cryopreservation for this group of patients.

Management in Early Pregnancy and Delivery

During pregnancy the woman infected with HBV or HCV should be followed up at the infectious disease department but can receive routine obstetric management.

The risk of infant HBV positivity at birth is unrelated to the method of delivery. Immediately after birth or at the latest within 48 hours, the child of an HBV-positive mother should receive HBV immunoglobulin and start vaccination against HBV. When the vaccination programme has been started, breastfeeding carries no risk of infecting the child.

Up to 5% of children born by HBV-positive mothers turn out to be infected despite the appropriate vaccination programme being carried out. Therefore it is recommended that all children born by HBV-positive mothers be tested for HBsAg and anti-HBs 1–2 months after the last vaccination.

If the woman is hepatitis C positive it is recommended not to use scalp electrodes during labour, but there is no specific contra-indication to vaginal delivery or breastfeeding. Transmission risk to a child during pregnancy/labour is low; however the child should be tested for HCV-RNA 6–12 months after birth.

Breastfeeding is not recommended if the infectious mother is on antiviral treatment.

Conclusion

Clinical practice in this area continues to be complicated by the lack of high-quality data regarding the precise risks of HBV and HCV transmission after IVF/ICSI treatment in hepatitis-discordant couples versus natural conception. Current approaches are therefore generally based on a "better-safe-than-sorry" principle. As more data become available and recommendations by national authorities develop, so will practice. Due to the complexity of the ART and the special information required by patients, it is our opinion that ART of viral-positive patients should be performed in specialized clinics in close collaboration with an infectious disease department.

Recommendations/Take-Home Message

1. Close contact with an infectious disease department is crucial.
2. Establish IVF procedures in collaboration with an infectious disease department and possibly with a local hygiene department.
3. Patients de novo detected positive for HBV or HCV at screening should be referred to an infectious disease department prior to onset of IVF treatment.
4. Partners of HBV-positive patients should be vaccinated prior to onset of IVF treatment.
5. IVF staff should be HBV vaccinated.
6. Semen washing with a double method is used to significantly reduce the viral load in the sperm fraction for use in IVF or ICSI.
7. Despite lack of evidence it seems best to use separate cryostorage for semen samples and embryos of HBV and HCV patients.

8. There remains a lack of data regarding the precise risks of HBV and HCV transmission after IVF/ICSI treatment in hepatitis-discordant couples versus natural conception.

REFERENCES

Bourlet T, Lornage J, Maertens A, Garret AS, Saoudin H, Tardy JC et al. Prospective evaluation of the threat related to the use of seminal fractions from hepatitis C virus-infected men in assisted reproductive techniques. *Hum Reprod.* 2009 Mar;24(3):530–5.

Chen H, Ge HS, Lv JQ, Wu XM, Xi HT, Huang JY, Zhu CF. Chronic hepatitis B virus infection in women is not associated with IVF/ICSI outcomes. *Arch Gynecol Obstet.* 2013 Jul 30. [Epub ahead of print]

Cobo A, Bellver J, de los Santos MJ, Remohí J. Viral screening of spent culture media and liquid nitrogen samples of oocytes and embryos from hepatitis B, hepatitis C, and human immunodeficiency virus chronically infected women undergoing *in vitro* fertilization cycles. *Fertil Steril.* 2012 Jan;97(1):74–8.

Englert Y, Moens E, Vannin AS, Liesnard C, Emiliani S, Delbaere A, Devreker F. Impaired ovarian stimulation during *in vitro* fertilization in women who are seropositive for hepatitis C virus and seronegative for human immunodeficiency virus. *Fertil Steril.* 2007 Sep;88(3):607–11. Epub 2007 Feb 22.

Foster GR. Past, present, and future hepatitis C treatments. *Semin Liver Dis.* 2004;24 Suppl 2:97–104.

Gerberding JL, Henderson DK. Management of occupational exposures to bloodborne pathogens: Hepatitis B virus, hepatitis C virus, and human immunodeficiency virus. *Clin Infect Dis.* 1992 Jun;14(6):1179–85.

Gilling-Smith C, Emiliani S, Almeida P, Liesnard C, Englert Y. Laboratory safety during assisted reproduction in patients with blood-borne viruses. *Hum Reprod.* 2005;20(6):1433–8.

Hanafi NF, Abo Ali AH, Aboelkheir HF. ICSI outcome in women who have positive PCR result for hepatitis C virus. *Hum Reprod.* 2011 Jan;26(1):143–7.

Hu XL, Zhou XP, Qian YL, Wu GY, Ye YH, Zhu YM. The presence and expression of the hepatitis B virus in human oocytes and embryos. *Hum Reprod.* 2011 Jul;26(7):1860–7.

Jonas MM. Hepatitis B and pregnancy: An underestimated issue. *Liver Int.* 2009;29:133–9.

Lam PM, Suen SH, Lao TT, Cheung LP, Leung TY, Haines C. Hepatitis B infection and outcomes of in vitro fertilization and embryo transfer treatment. *Fertil Steril.* 2010 Feb;93(2):480–5.

Lee VC, Ng EH, Yeung WS, Ho PC. Impact of positive hepatitis B surface antigen on the outcome of IVF treatment. *Reprod Biomed Online.* 2010 Nov;21(5):712–7.

Lutgens SP, Nelissen EC, van Loo IH, Koek GH, Derhaag JG, Dunselman GA. To do or not to do: IVF and ICSI in chronic hepatitis B virus carriers. *Hum Reprod.* 2009; 24:2676–8.

Nie R, Jin L, Zhang H, Xu B, Chen W, Zhu G. Presence of hepatitis B virus in oocytes and embryos: A risk of hepatitis B virus transmission during *in vitro* fertilization. *Fertil Steril.* 2011;95:1667–71.

NVOG (Dutch association for obstretrics and gynecology) position paper. http://nvog-documenten.nl/index.

Oger P, Yazbeck C, Gervais A, Dorphin B, Gout C, Jacquesson L et al. Adverse effects of hepatitis B virus on sperm motility and fertilization ability during IVF. *Reprod Biomed Online.* 2011 Aug;23(2):207–12.

Piratvisuth T. Optimal management of HBV infection during pregnancy. *Liver Int.* 2013 Feb;33 Suppl 1:188–94.

Söderström A, Norkrans G, Lindh M. Hepatitis B virus DNA during pregnancy and post partum: aspects on vertical transmission. *Scand J Infect Dis.* 2003;35(11–12):814–9.

Su H, Zhang Y, Xu D, Wang B, Zhang L, Li D, Xiao D, Li F, Zhang J, Yan Y. Occult hepatitis B virus infection in anti-HBs-positive infants born to HBsAg-positive mothers in China. *Plos One* 2013 Aug 12;8(8):e70768.

Tajiri H, Tanaka Y, Kagimoto S, Murakami J, Tokuhara D, Mizokami M. Molecular evidence of father-to-child transmission of hepatitis B virus. *J Med Virol.* 2007;79:922–6.

Tse KY, Ho LF, Lao T. The impact of maternal HBsAg carrier status on pregnancy outcomes: A case-control study. *J Hepatol.* 2005 Nov;43(5):771–5. Epub 2005 Jun 29.

Wingfield M, Cottell E. Viral screening of couples undergoing partner donation in assisted reproduction with regard to EU Directives 2004/23/EC, 2006/17/EC and 2006/86/EC: What is the evidence for repeated screening? *Hum Reprod.* 2010 Dec;25(12):3058–65.

Wong S, Chan LY, Yu V, Ho L. Hepatitis B carrier and perinatal outcome in singleton pregnancy. *Am J Perinatol.* 1999;16(9):485–8.

Zhou XP, Hu XL, Zhu YM, Qu F, Sun SJ, Qian YL. Comparison of semen quality and outcome of assisted reproductive techniques in Chinese men with and without hepatitis B. *Asian J Androl.* 2011 May;13(3):465–9.

18

The Couple Testing Positive for Human Immunodeficiency Virus

MV Sauer

CONTENTS

Introduction

Human immunodeficiency virus (HIV) infects nearly 35 million people worldwide. It affects women and men equally, although in the USA the majority of cases are found in reproductive-aged men.[1] Significant advancements in medical treatment using highly active antiretroviral therapy (HAART) have greatly improved survivorship, and for individuals compliant with therapy the illness is now considered a chronic ailment rather than a terminal disease. However, a diagnosis of HIV remains a devastating blow to an individual's expectations for a normal adult life. Couples in whom one or both partners are infected with HIV are often counselled against pregnancy for fear of both horizontal and vertical transmission of the virus.

Providing fertility care to couples in whom one or both partners is known to be HIV seropositive has been a subject of intense controversy.[2,3] Traditionally, reproductive options for HIV-serodiscordant or -seroconcordant couples have been limited. Donor sperm insemination and adoption represented the only recommended 'safe' options for the partners of HIV-seropositive men. However, reproductive drive is very strong, and patients are known to take unreasonable risks in order to have a baby. It is therefore not surprising that seroconversions of uninfected women occurred as a result of timed intercourse without a condom.

Impact of HIV Infection on IVF Outcomes

The impact of HIV on *in vitro* fertilization (IVF) per se is negligible. However, in general, patients who are HIV seropositive have not been granted access to fertility care. In side-by-side comparisons with HIV-seronegative men, men with HIV undergoing intracytoplasmic sperm injection (ICSI) have performed similarly with respect to fertilization in vitro, embryo quality, embryo implantation and pregnancy outcome.[4]

Impact of IVF on HIV Infection and Disease

Sperm washing with swim-up separates motile sperm from seminal plasma and non-motile cells (the compartment in which HIV resides). Success rates are largely dependent on factors that limit pregnancy outcomes for conventional patients undergoing infertility treatment, with the age of the female partner being the most significant prognostic indicator.[5] To date, there is no evidence to suggest that undergoing either IVF or intrauterine insemination (IUI) alters the course of the underlying disease.

IUI or IVF

There are advantages and disadvantages to using either IUI or IVF approaches. Although more cases of IUI have been reported, it remains unclear whether one approach is superior, and there are no randomized controlled trials to compare efficacy and safety.

IUI is technically easier, less expensive and, with repetitive applications, approaches the efficacy of IVF in well-selected patients. However, IUI therapy requires millions of sperm cells to be placed above the natural immunological barrier of the cervix. It is difficult to ensure that all lymphocytes and macrophages are eliminated from the 'washed' preparation. Since infection has been reported following IUI, and washed specimens may harbor virus, most centers recommend that all IUI specimens be tested for HIV prior to use. Viral testing adds complexity to the method and cost. Furthermore, men with chronic HIV infection often have abnormal semen profiles.[6] In such instances, IUI therapy may be less effective since pregnancy success is generally reduced in men with persistently abnormal semen analyses.

IVF with or without ICSI is commonly performed to treat male factor infertility and is available at centers providing assisted reproduction.[7] Similar to preparing sperm for IUI, discontinuous density gradient centrifugation techniques are utilized prior to IVF and ICSI, and only motile sperm found in the supernatant following swim-up are selected. Many fewer sperm are necessary for IVF, and typically fewer than 20 sperm are selected per case of IVF–ICSI.

There are also distinct disadvantages to IVF, as the cost is significantly greater in terms of both time and money. Patients undergo ovarian hyperstimulation prior to egg harvest, necessitating more monitoring. Oocyte aspiration is invasive and requires anesthesia. Ovarian hyperstimulation syndrome may occur, and multiple births further complicate many pregnancies.[8]

Preparing the Patient for IVF

HIV-infected patients should be under active medical surveillance for their illness by infectious disease specialists, and where appropriate, they should be prescribed antiviral medications. Plasma HIV RNA viral counts and CD4 status should be ascertained prior to beginning treatment. Table 18.1 lists recommendations and pretreatment tests performed prior to entry into our clinical program.

Partners should be HIV tested and be seronegative. Couples must remain compliant with safe sex practices and agree to use condoms. Women receive thorough pelvic examinations including Papanicolaou smears and cervical cultures, and serum estradiol, follicle-stimulating hormone (FSH) and anti-Mullerian hormone (AMH) levels are measured in order to evaluate the appropriateness of IVF therapy. HIV-seropositive women should receive prophylactic antibiotics prior to uterine cavity assessment (hysterosalpingography or sonohysterography), and medications should be extended for 7–10 days following the procedure to decrease the risk of post-procedure infection. Physicians should try to avoid examining HIV-seropositive women during their menstrual cycle to minimize blood contamination of examination rooms and ultrasound equipment. When blood is present, a thorough cleaning of exposed surfaces with a mild bleach solution is necessary to eradicate virus.

Managing the IVF Cycle

Standard protocols for ovarian hyperstimulation are prescribed. Needle aspiration of oocytes occurs 34–36 h following human chorionic gonadotropin (hCG) injection. A fresh semen sample is requested for IVF and ICSI. The use of semen preparation techniques, commonly referred to as 'sperm washing', has been recommended as a means of reducing the likelihood of horizontal transmission of HIV for over 20 years.[9] Results are encouraging, with reasonable pregnancy rates reported in more than 4000 published attempts and no seroconversions occurring in treated women or children.[10]

Most of this work has taken place in Europe, as there are few practitioners in the USA willing to offer therapy, presumably for fear of infecting the seronegative partner and child. The US Centers for Disease Control and Prevention (CDC) published recommendations against treating HIV-serodiscordant couples after HIV seroconversion occurred in a woman following IUI therapy with sperm from her HIV-seropositive husband.[11] Table 18.2 details the method used at Columbia University for sperm preparation.

Embryo transfers are typically scheduled on the third or fifth day. Assisted hatching of embryos and prophylactic steroids commonly prescribed at the time of embryo transfer are not used in HIV-seropositive patients.

Post-IVF Follow-Up

Serial blood testing (ultrasensitive HIV RNA polymerase chain reaction [PCR]) is repeated throughout pregnancy at the beginning of each trimester. At delivery and 3 months postpartum, mothers are tested using assays sensitive enough to detect virus

TABLE 18.1

Medical and Reproductive Pretreatment Recommendations and Tests

---

Female Patient

Age < 42 years

Day 2–3 FSH < 15 mIU/ml

Day 2–3 estradiol < 65 pg/ml

AMH > 0.17 ng/ml

Informed consent (risks, benefits and alternatives explained and documented)

Absence of opportunistic infections or prophylaxis

Infectious disease tests

  HIV-1 and HIV-2 (viral counts if HIV seropositive)

  Hepatitis A, B and C (HCV viral RNA counts if seropositive)

  Syphilis (RPR)

  Cervical cultures for gonorrhea and chlamydia

Hysterosalpingogram or saline infusion sonohysterogram (SIS)

Papanicolaou smear

Assessment of need for vaccinations

Genetic tests as appropriate

  Cystic fibrosis, hemoglobin electrophoresis, Tay–Sachs

Complete blood count (CBC) with platelets

CD4 counts (in HIV-seropositive women)

Thyroid-stimulating hormone (TSH)

SMA-12 with liver functions (in HIV- or HCV-infected women)

Blood type (Rh/ABO)

Medical clearance letter from internist dispensing HIV treatment

Medical clearance by maternal–fetal medicine

Male Patient

Semen analysis (if HIV or HCV seropositive must have adequate total motile count to perform
ICSI, typically > 1,000,000 motile sperm)

Infectious disease tests

  HIV-1 and HIV-2 (viral counts in seropositive men)

  Hepatitis A, B and C (HCV viral RNA counts in seropositive men)

  Syphilis (RPR)

Genetic tests

  Cystic fibrosis, hemoglobin electrophoresis, Tay–Sachs

Blood type (Rh/ABO)

CD4 counts (HIV-infected men)

Absence of opportunistic infections

Informed consent (risks, benefits and alternatives explained and documented)

SMA-12 and liver functions in HIV- and HCV-infected men

Medical clearance letter from internist dispensing HIV treatment

---

Note: AMH, anti-Mullerian hormone; FSH, follicle-stimulating hormone; HIV, human immunodeficiency virus; HCV, hepatitis C virus; RPR, rapid plasma reagin; SMA-12, sequential
multiple analysis (12-channel biochemical profile); Rh, rhesus; ICSI, intracytoplasmic
sperm injection.

TABLE 18.2

Semen Processing for *In Vitro* Fertilization–Intracytoplasmic Sperm Injection (IVF–ICSI)

Fresh semen sample collected at time of oocyte aspiration

Sample handled using strict sterile technique in a class II biological safety cabinet

Sample transferred to clean, sterile 15-ml centrifuge tube

Semen evaluated visually for sperm concentration, motility and extraneous cells

Semen centrifuged through a discontinuous density gradient as follows:

    1.5 ml of the lower (90%) layer pipetted into one (or more, depending on semen volume) tube

    1.5 ml of the upper (47%) layer carefully pipetted on top of this, and 1–2 ml of semen pipetted directly on top of the upper layer

    Gradient tube(s) centrifuged for 10–20 min at 300g

    Following spin, pellet(s) transferred to a clean tube and diluted with 5 ml of modified human tubal fluid (HTF) supplemented with 5% (v/v) human serum albumin (HSA)

    Sperm centrifuged for a maximum of 10 min at 300g and supernatant (wash number 1) removed

    Pellet resuspended in 3 ml of fresh modified HTF–HSA and spun again for a maximum of 5 min

    Supernatant (wash number 2) removed and the pellet resuspended in a small volume of modified HTF–HSA

    Sperm allowed 45-min period for 'swim-up'

Only sperm from final motile fraction selected for ICSI

TABLE 18.3

Clinical Results of the First 420 Consecutive Treatment Attempts Using *in vitro* Fertilization–Intracytoplasmic Sperm Injection (IVF–ICSI) in Human Immunodeficiency Virus Type 1 (HIV-1)-Serodiscordant Couples[12]

Number of couples treated	181
Number of initiated cycles	420
Number of attempts per couple	2.1 + 0.1 (1–6)
Cancellation rate due to poor ovarian response	15.8%
Number of oocytes aspirated per retrieval	15.0 + 0.5 (2–47)*
Number of fertilized oocytes per ICSI case	9.0 + 0.3 (0–24)*
Number of embryos transferred per attempt	3.0 + 0.1 (1–8)*
Percentage of couples with cryopreserved embryos	33.0%
Overall clinical pregnancy rate per embryo transfer	45.0%
Ongoing and delivered pregnancy rate per embryo transfer	37.0%
Cumulative pregnancy rate for couples over repeated attempts	80.4%
Number of seroconversions in treated women	0
Number of seroconversions in delivered offspring	0

* Mean ± SEM (range).

to the level of < 50 copies per ml of blood. Newborns are tested at birth and 3 months of age. Patients failing to become pregnant or women who experience spontaneous abortion are asked to repeat HIV tests 3 and 6 months later.

Table 18.3 details the initial 420 cycles of treatment in HIV-seropositive men.[12] Couples with fertility problems that are associated with poor IVF success rates should be counselled regarding their prognosis prior to undergoing treatment, given the unknown risk of HIV transmission that accompanies therapy.

The Special Needs of HIV-Seropositive Women

The prognosis for pregnant women with HIV has greatly improved with the introduction of HAART, which increases survival and enhances quality of life while reducing the risk of vertical transmission of HIV to the fetus from approximately 25% to < 2%.[13]

Many women with HIV desire to have children and seek professional help. In some cases the serodiscordant couple's fertility potential is presumed to be normal, and instruction on self-insemination may be all that is required. Often, other coexisting factors require medical assistance, particularly in cases of tubal disease. There remains little published experience relating to IVF services for HIV-seropositive women.[14]

Patient Selection and Methods of Treatment of HIV-Seropositive Women

Table 18.1 lists the requirements for HIV-seropositive women interested in participating in fertility services. Patients are commonly referred by consultants in infectious disease. Most require HAART to suppress HIV levels to low or preferably undetectable values.

Patients are given the option of self-insemination using semen collected in a sterile container by masturbation and drawn up into a 5-ml Bectin–Dickerson syringe for easy placement into the lower vagina. If women are discovered to have either tubal occlusion or severe abnormalities of their partner's semen then they are triaged to IVF–ICSI. IVF–ICSI is preferred to standard IVF in order to remove all adherent blood from the egg and surrounding cumulus.

Prior to beginning treatment, the patient's infectious disease consultant should attest to her clinical status and compliance with medications. Patients meet with a specialist in maternal–fetal medicine experienced with HIV. At this consultation, the management of the upcoming pregnancy, the need for careful surveillance for drug interactions and toxicity, and a plan for delivery and aftercare are reviewed. In women over the age of 35 years, chorionic villus sampling or amniocentesis is not recommended in order to minimize risk of infection in the fetus. Mothers do not breastfeed and receive bromocriptine postpartum to suppress lactation.

Additional Considerations

Women with HIV have unique needs and require subspecialty care to optimize outcomes. With respect to infectious disease, it is imperative that viral counts be maximally suppressed. Transmission risk to the fetus is known to correlate directly with HIV counts in the mother. The best results are in women with persistently low (<1000 copies) and preferably undetectable values. Certain medications, such as stavudine and efavirenz, are contraindicated for use during pregnancy, and in some cases adjustments to medications will be necessary prior to fertility treatment.[15]

Separate workstations and incubation and embryo storage facilities are necessary for handling the HIV-seropositive patient in order to minimize risk of viral contamination in the embryology laboratory. Pre-cycle consultation with anesthesiology is provided to review the drugs used during the aspiration.

All couples initially consult with a social worker and are encouraged to follow up for support during the pregnancy. The stigmatism of HIV infection often leads to isolation and depression. Substance abuse is also common, as patients self-medicate with alcohol or drugs. It is essential to the success of any program that ongoing systems be in place to evaluate and treat psychosocial disorders.

The Evolving Role of Pre-Exposure Prophylaxis and Physician-Assisted Fertility Care

Pre-exposure prophylaxis (PrEP) refers to the use of topical or oral antiretroviral therapy to reduce the risk of HIV transmission to uninfected individuals during sexual intercourse. The efficacy of daily administration of PrEP in reducing the risk of infection has been demonstrated in randomized controlled trials among HIV-serodiscordant men and women.[16] It also was employed in a well-designed observational clinical trial reported in 2011 in which pregnancy rates with timed intercourse paralleled those normally seen following the more complicated IUI with swim-up methods.[17] However, candidates for this approach must be very carefully selected, screened and followed in order to minimize transmission risk.

At Columbia University PrEP is offered in combination with IUI and swim-up with fresh untested specimens in couples in which the male has demonstrated undetectable viral loads in his serum for at least 6 months, is under the active care of an infectious disease specialist, and has a normal semen analysis. The female partner must have patent fallopian tubes and be willing to take PrEP from the time of the luteinizing hormone (LH) surge and continued for an additional 2 days (total 3 days). After 6 unsuccessful attempts couples should be re-evaluated and consideration for IVF be entertained to reduce cumulative exposure to infectious risk.

Summary of Management Options

It remains to be seen whether health-care providers in the field of assisted reproduction embrace the HIV-infected patient. Despite statements by the American Society for Reproductive Medicine,[16] the American College of Obstetricians and Gynecologists[17] and the European Society of Human Reproduction and Embryology[18] encouraging physicians to provide care to HIV-seropositive men and women, few programs are known to be openly compliant. Although patients cannot be discriminated against under US law and are protected by the Americans with Disability Act,[19] caregivers often claim conscientious-objector status and refer patients to programs that accept and treat. In our experience, the integration of HIV-infected patients into our clinical practice has not created undue hardships. Collaboration with infectious disease, maternal–fetal medicine, pediatrics and social services provides patients with a unique highly focused and specialized team of health-care providers to attend to their multiple needs and the needs of their baby. This unusually high level of surveillance positively reinforces the importance of compliance with medicines and physician directives.

The purpose of all clinical trials involving assisted reproduction is to provide HIV-serodiscordant couples with an opportunity to have a child without risk of viral transmission. Various techniques have been suggested as preventive measures to avoid infection in HIV-serodiscordant couples intent on reproducing. The commonly accepted principles of health-care ethics include consideration of respect for autonomy, non-maleficence, beneficence, fidelity and justice.[20] Each of these tenets should be individually considered in deciding whether or not to treat. Informed and rational decision-making must occur in every case of intervention. A lengthy discussion of the natural history of HIV infection, and the biology of transmission, should precede treatment. Alternatives, including artificial insemination with donor sperm, adoption and childless living, should also be offered. A balanced and non-prejudicial view towards treatment is requisite, and typically mandates that professionals outside the IVF team be involved. Patients must act intentionally and without controlling a free and voluntary act. Most important, women need to understand that no procedure is risk free, and all carry a small possibility for infection in themselves and their babies.

REFERENCES

1. Centers for Disease Control and Prevention. Estimated HIV incidence among adults and adolescents in the United States, 2007–2010. *HIV Surveillance Supplemental Report* 2012;17(No. 4), http://www.cdc.gov/hiv/topics/surveillance/resources/reports/#supplemental. December 2012.
2. Englert Y, Van Vooren JP, Place I, et al. ART in HIV-infected couples. Has the time come for a change in attitude? *Hum Reprod* 2001; 16: 1309–15.
3. Sauer MV. American physicians remain slow to embrace the reproductive needs of human immunodeficiency virus-infected patients. *Fertil Steril* 2006; 85: 295–7.
4. Sauer MV, Chang PL. Establishing a program to assist HIV-1 seropositive men to have children using IVF–ICSI. *Am J Obstet Gynecol* 2002; 186: 627–33.
5. Chu MC, Pena JE, Thornton MH, et al. Assessing the efficacy of IVF and ICSI in HIV-1 serodiscordant couples. *Reprod Biomed Online* 2005; 10: 130–4.
6. Gilling-Smith C, Frodsham LCG, Tamberlin B, et al. Reducing reproductive risks in HIV infected couples: A comprehensive programme of care. *Hum Reprod* 2003; 18: 581–7.
7. Dale B, Elder K, editors. Micromanipulation techniques. In *In Vitro Fertilization*. Cambridge: Cambridge University Press, 1997: 150–76.
8. Pena JE, Thornton MH, Sauer MV. Complications of IVF–ICSI in HIV serodiscordant couples. *Arch Gynecol Obstet* 2003; 268: 198–201.
9. Semprini AE, Levi-Setti P, Bozzo M, et al. Insemination of HIV-negative women with processed semen of HIV-positive partners. *Lancet* 1992; 340: 1317–19.
10. Vitorino RL, Grinsztejn BG, Ferreira de Andrade CA, Hokerberg YHM, Veira de Souza CT, Friedman RK, Passos SRL. Systematic review of the effectiveness and safety of assisted reproduction techniques in couples serodiscordant for human immunodeficiency virus where the man is positive. *Fertil Steril* 2011; 95: 1684–90.
11. HIV-1 infection and artificial insemination with processed semen. *MMWR Morbid Mortal Weekly Rep* 1990; 39: 249, 255–6.
12. Sauer MV, Wang JG, Douglas NC, Nakhuda GS, Vardhana P, Jovanovic V, Guarnaccia MM. Providing fertility care to men seropositive for human immunodeficiency virus: Reviewing 10 years of experience and 420 consecutive cycles of *in vitro* fertilization and intracytoplasmic sperm injection. *Fertil Steril* 2009; 91: 2455–60.
13. Townsend CL, Cortina-Borja M, Peckham CS, de Ruiter A, Lyall H, Tookey PA. Low rates of mother-to-child transmission of HIV following effective pregnancy interventions in the United Kingdom and Ireland, 2000–2006. *AIDS* 2008; 22: 973–81.

14. Nurudeen SK, Grossman LC, Bourne L, Guarnaccia MM, Sauer MV, Douglas NC. Reproductive outcomes of HIV seropositive women treated by assisted reproduction. *J Womens Health* 2013; 22: 243–9.

15. Douglas NC, Wang JG, Yu B, Gaddipati S, Guarnaccia MM, Sauer MV. A systematic, multidisciplinary approach to address the reproductive needs of HIV-seropositive women. *Reprod Biomed Online* 2009; 19: 257–63.

16. Baeten JM, Donnell D, Ndase P, et al. Antiretroviral prophylaxis for HIV prevention in heterosexual men and women. *N Engl J Med* 2012; 367: 399–410.

17. Vernazza PL, Graf I, Sonnenberg-Schwan U, Geit M, Meurer A. Preexposure prophylaxis and time intercourse for HIV-discordant couples willing to conceive a child. *AIDS* 2011; 25: 2005–2008.

18. Ethics Committee of the ASRM. HIV and infertility treatment. *Fertil Steril* 2002; 77: 218–22.

19. American College of Obstetricians and Gynecologists. HIV: Ethical Guidelines for Obstetricians and Gynecologists, April 2001. ACOG Committee Opinion 255. Washington, DC: ACOG, 2001.

20. The ESHRE Ethics and Law Task Force. Task Force 8: Ethics of medically assisted fertility treatment for HIV positive men and women. *Hum Reprod* 2004; 19: 2454–6.

21. Annas GJ. Protecting patients from discrimination – the Americans with Disabilities Act and HIV infection. *N Engl J Med* 1998; 339: 1255–9.

22. Sauer MV. Providing assisted reproductive care to HIV-serodiscordant couples: Time to re-examine healthcare policy. *Am J Bioethics* 2003; 3: 33–40.

19

The Couple with Sexual Dysfunction

WL Gianotten

CONTENTS

KEY WORDS: *vaginismus, post-traumatic stress disorder (PTSD), anejaculation, vibrator, self-management, sexual dysfunction*

Introduction

Whereas sexual dysfunction can interfere with natural conception, not conceiving can interfere with pleasurable sex and sexual function. Although in the process of assisted reproduction technologies (ARTs) the pleasure element becomes less important, other aspects of sexual functioning become increasingly important. In that process, producing sperm at the right time and allowing invasive vaginal procedures such as vaginal ultrasound and speculum introduction become vital. This chapter looks at various types of sexual dysfunction that can interfere with the outcome of ART and in vitro fertilization (IVF). In addition, attention is paid to possible long-term emotional and sexual side effects of these fertility interventions.

Impact of Sexual Dysfunction on the IVF Procedure and Outcome

Sexual dysfunction can disturb the process of IVF. Low desire in the man can cause low arousal with difficulties to keep an erection and subsequently to ejaculate. Erectile dysfunction (ED) does not interfere with IVF, but can complicate orgasm/ejaculation. Some causes for ED are related to the wish to conceive, and this may be manifest as performance failure caused by the high pressure to produce sperm on demand. In other men ED is related to ambivalence about a pregnancy. Clearly, male ejaculation is necessary for conception. Some cases of orgasm dysfunction (OD) are caused by ambivalence regarding pregnancy. Other men have OD only during intercourse, but not when masturbating. Lifelong anejaculation, usually resulting from a combination of character- and religious-based sexual inhibitions, is more difficult to overcome during IVF treatment.

Vaginismus is regularly found in the population with an unfulfilled wish to conceive. Many of these couples only have intercourse to become pregnant. However the vaginismus can seriously hamper intravaginal procedures. Together, these elements may result in the wish to conceive by IVF providing the motivation to accept treatment for vaginismus.

Post-traumatic stress disorder (PTSD) due to sexual abuse is not always sufficiently investigated and treated prior to embarking on IVF treatment. PTSD can cause sudden emotional breakdown in situations resembling the former sexual abuse situation. The stress of IVF combined with pelvic examination may create such circumstances.

Impact of IVF on Sexuality

Before commencing IVF treatment, in some couples the challenge of facing infertility may already have compromised sexuality and sexual function. Failure to conceive is often a blow to female and male identity, causing low desire. Ovulation-based timing of intercourse reduces sexual desire and arousal, potentially causing female dyspareunia. Subsequent medical interventions may further the decline in sexual quality. Spontaneity disappears when timing and orgasm are dictated by physician or treatment protocol. In some men, the expectation to sexually perform at predetermined times can increase stress. Sexual intimacy may be reduced by (repeated) genital examination and by having to share details of sexual activities.

The sexual relationship itself can therefore also become stressed. One or both partners may feel irritation as a result of the tension and disappointment or by the message that one of them is the cause of the infertility. Moreover, mutual contact will diminish because male and female tend to react differently to the practical challenges and the emotional effects of stress on the sexual relationship.

The more the fertility treatment invades the couple's physical and emotional privacy, the further sexual desire will be reduced, increasingly damaging the sexual relationship. Sexual function and pleasure are frequently disturbed in patients awaiting ART, and around 25% have been reported to suffer from related depression.[1] In some women the pain or perceived pain of vaginal procedures will trigger an already tense hypertonic pelvic floor, resulting in a complete 'closing' of the vagina.

When women have a history of sexual or physical abuse that has received insufficient attention, various aspects of the fertility treatment can cause violent flashbacks (re-experiencing traumas). Since this can seriously interfere with the procedure, the possibility of previous abuse should be investigated before commencing IVF treatment.

Men are in their own way sensitive to the stress of infertility and IVF. The diagnosis of infertility can shatter male self-esteem, and it has been reported that 10% of men develop sexual dysfunction following a diagnosis of infertility. There is some evidence that emotional stress of an IVF program can negatively affect the quality of semen.[2] Moreover, the 'superstress' of the moment with the necessity to perform may depress sexual performance, expressing itself as erectile or orgasmic failure.

Preparing the Patient for IVF

Careful history taking is an important tool in preparation and prevention of problems. Poor male sexual functioning, with imminent or real ED or OD, should instigate the investigation of thorough differential diagnosis. In case of performance failure due to the stress of the moment, additional (sexological) counselling should be considered, and the potential benefits of backup procedures (such as availability of freezing sperm before the day it is required) and pharmacological and visual erotic support should be explained and offered. However, when ambivalence towards fatherhood or the relationship itself affects sexual function, the decision to proceed with ART should be reconsidered.

Any major sexual dysfunction that strongly will reduce the chance of spontaneous conception should be addressed before entering IVF treatment. Such an approach will prevent additional emotional damage to the couple and reduce frustration for the medical team.

Often it will be possible to reduce the stress arising from other sexual dysfunctions by explaining the impact of stress and offering backup procedures. When counselling was offered in an IVF program setting, the semen quality of the vast majority of patients did not appear to be significantly affected by the stress of participation on the day of oocyte recovery.[3]

Previous sexual or physical abuse can cause violent flashbacks and seriously disturb various elements of the IVF procedure, and this area therefore merits investigation prior to embarking with treatment by ART. When sexual violence has not yet been sufficiently addressed, a thorough assessment is needed by a psychiatrist or psychotherapist with (sexual) trauma expertise.

There is considerable individual variation in the long-term consequences of sexual (or physical) trauma. On the less-severe side (usually the result of a single event) a relatively short treatment process may be all that is required for dealing with the aftermath. In the more severe cases (usually after chronic or repeated abuse exposure) PTSD includes abuse-related alterations in brain functioning with increased vulnerability to stress. In such cases, it is recommended to delay fertility treatment. ART should not be started without counselling by an experienced therapist, who can also address the practical aspects of the various procedures.

In the most severe cases it is strongly recommended to reconsider the request to conceive by IVF, or indeed whether it is wise for the couple to conceive at all. Not being survivors, but victims, these women may never be able to develop a good enough relationship with a child.[4,5]

When expecting superstress in the woman as a result of insufficiently resolved vaginismus or sexual violence, additional preparation is needed. In such situations it is advisable to build a relationship based on trust with one professional who will be present at every procedure. Usually this will be a female (although if the abuser was female, a male may be needed).

This approach may also be extended to having all vaginal interventions performed by one trusted member of the fertility team. In other cases the process can be facilitated when the woman is counselled by a female psychosomatic professional who can advise beforehand how to handle the stress, who recognizes the patient's reaction pattern and who will be present during all procedures. For some women, the partner can have that role. Being conscious of having control over process and interventions can prevent emotional breakdown in some of these women. One way to have control is for the patient to be allowed to insert the speculum or vaginal ultrasound probe herself.

First Do No Harm

Modern techniques make it possible to minimize the sexually confrontational aspects of IVF. Harvesting sperm by epididymal aspiration and transferring the embryo can be done under general anesthesia. That, however, is not always wise. A strong urge to conceive can blind couples to the potential damage of fertility interventions. Some couples may focus purely on achieving a pregnancy by 'quick fix', whereas a longer-term approach to solving sexual problems may result not only in pregnancy but also in other relational benefits. The anorgasmic man who 'loses' half a year undergoing treatment, but then can ejaculate by himself will probably be much happier in the longer term than the man who underwent epididymal aspiration. Similarly, the woman with PTSD who loses a year to treatment but then is able to undergo the procedures fully conscious, without loss of control, may be much happier and less damaged than the woman who becomes pregnant through vaginal procedures under general anesthesia.

The quick fix that some couples seek for their fertility problem is more likely to exacerbate rather than help the couple's sexual problems. Our aim should be to minimize these negative effects. After all, the final target is a happy family with happy parenthood. Less stress and a more satisfying sexual life will keep the relationship in better order, and accordingly benefit the relation of both parents with the new child.[6]

Some subfertile couples may therefore be best advised to invest in a period with regular intercourse (several times a week) and better-quality sex (with good arousal, ample time to ejaculation, not too long an interval between ejaculations, and no use of lubricants). This will also maximize the chance to conceive should ART be unsuccessful.[7]

Managing the IVF Cycle

The key problems which need to be addressed in the context of managing the IVF cycle are erectile problems, ejaculation problems, vaginismus and PTSD.

Erectile Dysfunction

In ART, ED must be taken seriously since diminished sexual excitement can disturb ejaculation. This can be a good indication to prescribe one of the phosphodiesterase-5 (PDE5) inhibitors, which should be taken approximately one hour before masturbation. Explicit discussion is recommended, allowing other strategies for achieving sexual stimulation to enhance excitement and erection to be considered. These may include presence of the partner; use of fantasies; sexually explicit audiovisuals or magazines. Most men are sensitive to visual sexual stimulation, especially moving pictures. They are obviously facilitating factors when the man 'has to' produce semen.[8] Since most men will know what turns them on, they should be advised to use that (and eventually bring their own X-rated material). The fertility unit obviously should have a room for masturbation; with a proper erotic environment; proper audiovisual facilities and where the man (or couple) can be assured they will not be disturbed. Many men will find it embarrassing to request erotic material, so it should automatically be available in the room or provided routinely to every man.

Retrograde Ejaculation

Retrograde ejaculation (RE) impairs sperm quality and complicates the clinical process. Pharmacological treatment, as the least-invasive option, should be tried first. Imipramine, chlorpheniramine and phenylpropanalamine show the best reversal rates in RE.[9] In spinal-cord injured men usually vibration is needed. A silicone balloon catheter can be employed to tamponade the bladder neck for antegrade ejaculation without urine contamination.[10] Alternatively, sperm can be retrieved from urine produced after masturbation.

Anejaculation

The majority of men with anejaculation will fit within four groups based on anejaculation cause: neurological damage; medication induced; lifelong emotionally inhibited and situational (performance failure).

Due to Neurological Damage

Over 80% of young men suffering from spinal cord injury can ejaculate with strong penile vibratory stimulation. An effective approach is to use the FertiCare® vibrator, at a frequency of 100 Hz and a peak-to-peak amplitude of 2.5 mm, with rectal electroejaculation reserved for failures.[11] Recently non-spinal cord injury patients have been shown to benefit from the use of midodrine.[12]

Medication Induced

A high percentage of OD is a well-known side effect of antidepressants, with selective serotonin reuptake inhibitors (SSRIs) and venlafaxine most notorious. Half of the men on this medication cannot ejaculate. Various strategies can be used to 're-induce' orgasm/ejaculation. The serotonin changes can be counteracted with antidotes, for example antiserotonergic cyproheptadine (4–16 mg, 1 h before intercourse or masturbation) or dopaminergic amantadine. Other recommended antidotes are bupropion (150 mg, 3 h before), methylphenidate (5 mg, 1 h before) and sildenafil (100 mg, 1 h before). In the case of SSRIs with a short half-life, the serotonergic action can be counteracted by not taking the drug for 72 h. Sexual function will then have returned to near normal in most men, usually without impairment of the antidepressive or anti-anxiety action. When this strategy with paroxetine causes symptoms of acute withdrawal, halving the dose for 72 h can be tried. The 'drug holiday' strategy cannot be used with fluoxetine because of the long half-life.

Any approach should be topped up by proper stimulation (visual, vibration, etc.).

Lifelong Emotionally Inhibited

Because it is lifelong, emotional inhibition is poorly amenable to acute treatment. However, with properly applied treatment the results are reasonable. To avoid more invasive procedures such as electroejaculation or testis biopsy one could try to harvest and cryopreserve the nocturnal emission. This usually happens more easily after 'sexual priming' (administering before sleep as much erotic stimulation as is acceptable). Some of these men learn to ejaculate with a strong vibrator (FertiCare®), eventually combined with pharmacologic support. Although there is some clinical experience with antiserotonergics (cyproheptadine), dopaminergics (amantadine) and stimulants (methylphenidate), convincingly effective treatments are not yet available. Midodrine could be another option.[12] It is obvious that one should aim at both relaxation ('let it go') and sexual excitement. However, in practice many of these men are not amenable to the use of erotic imagination, visual stimulation, etc.

Situational

In the situational case, the man fails to ejaculate because of the stress of the moment. The approach basically consists of diminishing the insecurity and performance failure and increasing the stimulation. Insecurity can be partially reduced by information on backup solutions ("If you don't succeed, don't worry; we have several other solutions!"). For instance, having a cryopreserved sperm sample (even if the quality is not that good) can diminish the performance failure. Stimulation can be increased by combining the use of a PDE5 inhibitor for maintaining erection, a vibrator and visually explicit erotic stimulation.

Poor Ejaculate

When the ejaculate is of poor quality one can try to improve this on the day of oocyte pickup. High sexual stimulation during masturbation with X-rated videos has been shown to result in recovery of spermatozoa of greater fertilizing potential in both normozoospermic and cryptozoospermic men.[13] This sometimes can obviate the need for testicular biopsy. Another way to enhance the ejaculate quality is extending the excitement phase. The duration of pre-ejaculatory sexual arousal is an important predictor of ejaculate quality for specimens produced by masturbation.[14] This can be troublesome in busy departments. A quiet room, well adapted for this masturbation purpose, could diminish the stress for both the men and the department.

Vaginismus

For many couples wishing to conceive, vaginismus is no longer a problem when they realise that it can be solved by self-insemination. However when vaginal ultrasound, intrauterine insemination or embryo transfer is inevitable, vaginismus becomes a major obstacle. Obviously it is best to treat the vaginismus before ART is started.

Unfortunately, fertility departments regularly are caught in the 'catch 22' situation where treatment is promised or already started and the woman's vaginismus threatens to disturb the process. What strategies can be employed to overcome this?

General Anaesthesia

The seemingly logical solution of general anaesthesia is very threatening to many women with vaginismus. The clinical experience is that the anxiety goes up and the 'vaginistic behavior' is prolonged because of the loss of control.

Self-Hypnosis, Self-Relaxation and Imagery

Self-hypnosis techniques usually can be learned in a short period of time. The woman learns induction, then deepening and then proceeding to 'a safe place'. Self-relaxation training can include progressive muscle relaxation with elements of meditation. Improving the positive imagery capacities is another way of coping with pain and other threatening moments. These strategies can be combined with self-management.

Self-Management

Having control over the situation can be the key to self-management. For some women, a feeling of self-competence is more important than a bit of pain. Many women can learn to introduce the speculum or vaginal probe herself. This is easier when she is always attended by the same fertility professionals.

Medication

While psychiatrists have tried anxiolytics and gynaecologists have tried general muscle relaxants, none of these medications has been shown to be effective in helping women in the resolution of their vaginismus. Losing control under medication can be a threatening experience.

A new strategy is the use of botulinum toxin.[15] Usually under anaesthesia, the drug is injected in or around the muscles of the pelvic floor, eventually followed by progressive vaginal dilation. It prevents 'closing the vagina', at least on pelvic floor level. This apparently helps in women with 'defloration phobia', who are brought up with much fear for pain and bleeding in cultures with high value for virginity, because their problem has disappeared after the first intercourse. In the Western world many cases of vaginismus are *penetration phobia* (where in some of the women the disturbance also continues after the first intercourse).

The Aftermath of Trauma and Post-Traumatic Stress Disorder

When harbouring memories of sexual trauma, the vaginal interventions of ART can be very threatening. The combination of being undressed, lying down, having someone standing between her legs (especially when male), experiencing the stress of the situation ("Will I become pregnant?"), having items inserted in her vagina and eventually suffering pain can cause vivid flashbacks and memories. With the patient anxious, screaming or crying, with the husband confused or angry and with the physician confused, angry and maybe guilty, one could call this an acute emergency. Such situations should be prevented. Unfortunately, there is no quick-fix approach such as general anaesthesia or anxiolytics since they will be experienced as revictimisation because of losing control again. Being aware of traumatic histories, it is best to put treatment strategies in place prior to intervention. However, one cannot always wait until that process is complete. In many cases patients do not need a full trauma treatment and can learn within a short treatment to handle the stress of ART. So what can be done?

Treatment Strategies

Not losing control is a most important principle here. Ahead of the intervention the woman should know exactly what will happen, and she should be allowed (as far as feasible) to have control during the various steps of the procedure, for example by saying 'Stop'. Dealing with this technique has to be learned also by the physician and the other members of the team. With these patients in particular, the professional should always be the same person and preferably female. On some moments of the process, control is not feasible, and the patient should be prepared and learn how to handle the emotions that may surface during such temporary lack of control. During this explanation and learning stage she should again and again be able to reconsider her decision. Depending on the seriousness of the emotional disturbance this counselling and developing of skills to deal with the intervention can be done by a therapist, by a fertility nurse or by the physician. Depending on his emotional capacities, the partner should be used since his (or her) support and expertise dealing with the patient's emotions can be very helpful.

Tools that may be useful for preparing women to undergo these interventions are self-hypnosis ('going to a safe place'), imagery exercises, relaxation exercises (breathing exercises), and using meditation music and transitional objects (like a cuddly toy) that help the woman feel that this time no harm will be done to her.

The sense of control can be increased when the woman or her partner can carry out part of the procedure as described in vaginismus (such as self-introducing speculum or probe).

Medication

Medication is regularly used in the course of a full PTSD treatment to relax the patient sufficiently so that she can pass through the psychotherapy process. In the clinical context of ART an anxiolytic with retrograde amnesic actions may be helpful in reducing stress. Unfortunately, however, this strategy usually diminishes the sense of control. Medication may numb the woman's body or disconnect her from her body. The situation becomes more tricky in the woman who experienced dissociation during her abuse because this comes close to re-creating the abuse. It becomes plainly disastrous in the woman who has been doped during her abuse. Hence medication frequently is inappropriate.

There are, however, patients for whom medication can be helpful. Some women have learned to use a fast-acting anxiolytic when starting to feel anxious. That experience should become integrated in the counselling in a way that the woman knows to be in control of that medication, and if and when to use it. In an integrated approach some women benefit from learning how to use and handle their own anxiolytic. Using an unknown preparation is far more risky.

In Acute Emergencies

In the course of the procedure the patient can collapse emotionally. What should be done when it suddenly really goes wrong? Depending on the situation, one has to decide the best strategy: administer a strong anxiolytic and continue the procedure; stop the procedure and try to calm the woman before continuing; or announce stopping the procedure completely. Usually the partner will know how best to calm the patient, for example by the partner or a nurse holding the patient. Whatever strategy is followed, afterwards ample time and attention should be devoted to sort out exactly what happened, how to proceed and eventually how this can be prevented next time.

Post-IVF Follow-Up

Optimal continuation of the sexual relationship deserves attention, especially when ART has contributed to a disturbed sexual life. For couples leaving treatment without a child, regained sex and intimacy can be the vital element in continuing their relationship. For couples who conceive and become parents, sex and intimacy will be needed both to preserve the 'lover' aspects of their relationship and to cope with the hassles of young parenthood. It should be clear that inquiring about the condition of the sexual life and explaining about the importance of regaining sexual intimacy are relevant aspects of care. In the case of problems, referral to an experienced sex therapist or sexual medicine professional should be offered.

Summary of Management Options

1. Be aware that in assisted reproduction, the procreative aspects of sex can easily harm or even destroy the recreational and the relationship aspects of sex and as such, the quality of life.
2. Give attention to sexual history taking as this will aid in anticipating the various reactions to the stress of ART, such as ejaculatory performance failure and re-experienced sexual abuse.

3. In the case of erectile or ejaculatory failure, spend time motivating the man as much as possible into maximum sexual stimulation (vibrator, X-rated movies, PDE5 inhibitor, etc.).

4. Ensure that the fertility unit has a room optimally equipped and maintained for masturbation with vibrator and visual stimulation available, where the man (or the couple) can spend time without being disturbed.

5. In the case of a history of insufficiently addressed sexual abuse, ask for assessment by a professional experienced in dealing with sexual violence. If possible, put treatment strategies in place prior to intervention.

6. In the case of vaginismus (and sexual abuse experience), spend time during preparation on self-management strategies and let all procedures be done by the same team.

7. In the case of a history of sexual abuse (when keeping control is very important for the woman), ensure counselling and preparation for both the couple and the team on how to handle the stress of the situation. Use anxiolytic medication only within such a combined approach.

REFERENCES

1. Oddens BJ, Tonkelaar den I, Nieuwenhuyse H. Psychosocial problems in women facing fertility problems. *Hum Reprod* 1999;13:255–61.
2. Ragni G, Caccamo A. Negative effect of stress of *in vitro* fertilization program on quality of semen. *Acta Eur Fertil* 1992;23:21–3.
3. Drudy L, Harrison R, Verso J, et al. Does patient semen quality alter during an *in vitro* fertilization (IVF) program in a manner that is clinically significant when specific counseling is in operation? *J Assist Reprod Genet* 1994;11:185–8.
4. Trickett PK, Noll JG, Putnam FW. The impact of sexual abuse on female development: Lessons from a multigenerational, longitudinal research study. *Dev Psychopathol* 2011;23:453–76.
5. Cohen T. Motherhood among incest survivors. *Child Abuse Negl* 1995;19:1423–9.
6. von Sydow K. Sexuality during pregnancy and after childbirth: A metacontent analysis of 59 studies. *J Psychosom Res* 1999;47:27–49.
7. Stanford JB, Mikolajczyk RT, Lynch CD, et al. Cumulative pregnancy probabilities among couples with subfertility: Effects of varying treatments. *Fertil Steril* 2010;93:2175–81.
8. van Roijen JH, Slob AK, Gianotten WL, et al. Sexual arousal and the quality of semen produced by masturbation. *Hum Reprod* 1996;11:147–51.
9. Kamischke A, Nieschlag E. Update on medical treatment of ejaculatory disorders. *Int J Andro* 2002;25:333–44.
10. Lim TC, Mallidis C, Hill ST, et al. A simple technique to prevent retrograde ejaculation during assisted ejaculation. *Paraplegia* 1994;32:142–9.
11. Ohl DA, Sonksen J, Menge AC, et al. Electroejaculation versus vibratory stimulation in spinal cord injured men: Sperm quality and patient preference. *J Urol* 1997;157:2147–9.
12. Safarinejad MR. Midodrine for the treatment of organic anejaculation but not spinal cord injury: A prospective randomized placebo-controlled double-blind clinical study. *Int J Impot Res* 2009;21:213–20.

13. Yamamoto Y, Sofikitis N, Mio Y, et al. Influence of sexual stimulation on sperm parameters in semen samples collected via masturbation from normozoospermic men or cryptozoospermic men participating in an assisted reproduction programme. *Andrologia* 2000;32(3):131–8.
14. Pound N, Javed MH, Ruberto C, et al. Duration of sexual arousal predicts semen parameters for masturbatory ejaculates. *Physiol Behav* 2002;76:685–9.
15. Pacik PT. Vaginismus: review of current concepts and treatment using botox injections, bupivacaine injections, and progressive dilation with the patient under anesthesia. *Aesthetic Plast Surg* 2011;35:1160–4.

20

The IVF Patient, International Travel and Vaccinations

H Tijani and NS Macklon

CONTENTS

Introduction

Global travel trends have increased over the years and increasingly involve journeys to remote parts of the world. The World Health Organisation (WHO) has estimated that more than 900 million international journeys are undertaken every year.[1] It is therefore clear that increasing numbers of people in the *in vitro* fertilisation (IVF) population are undertaking international travel and are likely to seek advice from professionals beforehand. While it is generally advisable that IVF patients should defer travel until the outcome of treatment is known, when travel is necessary in the period preceding, during or following IVF treatment, a number of issues should be discussed and managed appropriately. These include the risks associated with long-haul flights, such as deep venous thrombosis (DVT; see Chapter 2); the risk of sustaining complications from an early pregnancy loss or ectopic pregnancy; dealing with the physical, emotional and psychological stress from subfertility and treatment; and the risks and benefits of vaccination against disease.

TABLE 20.1

Estimate of Risks of Requiring Healthcare when Travelling Abroad

For those travelling to a developing country for 1 month:

50% will develop a health problem during their trip.

8% will see a doctor.

5% will be sufficiently ill to have to stay in bed.

0.3% will require hospital admission (either abroad or on return).

0.05% will require air evacuation.

0.001% will die.

Only 1–4% of travel-related deaths are due to infectious disease. Injury, usually due to road traffic accidents (RTAs), is the most common cause of mortality and morbidity.

Source: Adapted from Spira AM. *Lancet.* 2003 Apr 19; 361(9366):1368–81. With permission.

Pre-Travel Evaluation

Table 20.1 summarises the general risks of encountering health problems when travelling abroad.[2] An IVF patient contemplating travelling should be encouraged to consult a healthcare professional/travel clinic. Ideally, it should be a face-to-face consultation, preferably with input from the woman's fertility specialist to enable risk and advice to be individualised and the best package of preventive measures to be put in place. If the woman is pregnant, it may be appropriate to seek advice from an obstetrician, particularly if there are additional medical complications.

The pre-travel evaluation of the IVF patient should begin with a medical history, with particular attention to assessing how the risks associated with IVF such as ovarian hyperstimulation syndrome (OHSS) and early pregnancy problems may affect the risks of travel. A review of the patient's travel itinerary, including destinations, types of accommodation, and planned activities, should guide pre-travel health advice. Checking for immunity to various infectious diseases may obviate the need for some vaccines.

Preparation should also include educating the patient regarding avoidance of travel-associated risks with poor hygiene or diet and recognition of more serious complications. Feeling bloated, abdominal pain, nausea, vomiting, shortness of breath and bleeding are conditions that require urgent medical attention.

A systematic approach to the risk assessment and management should be employed such as the one in Table 20.2.

When Is It Safe to Travel?

Little evidence is available as to what constitute absolute contraindications to travel in the IVF patient. However, women with certain medical conditions should be advised against travelling, and this decision will need to be made on an individual basis, after discussion with the relevant medical specialist(s).

TABLE 20.2

Pre-Travel Consultation Checklist for the IVF Patient Traveller

- Assess: general health/background medical conditions
  - specific issues: stage of IVF treatment
    - ensure potential problems are identified/excluded (e.g. OHSS, miscarriage, ectopic pregnancy, etc.)
- Vaccination status: check immunity to infectious diseases (e.g. hepatitis A and B, rubella, varicella, measles, pertussis)
- Vaccination requirements: update routine immunizations: tetanus-diphtheria-pertussis, influenza (inactivated), polio, including hepatitis A and B
- Destination risk assessment
  - malaria
  - infectious diseases: vector-, air-, blood-, food- and water-borne risks
    - outbreak of disease requiring a live virus vaccine
    - outbreak of a disease for which no vaccine is available but which has a high risk of maternal or fetal illness or death
  - environmental: altitude, heat, humidity,
  - medical services available during transit and at destination
- Travel risk assessment
  - mode of travel, destination, length of travel
  - purpose of travel: holiday, visiting friends and relatives, pilgrimage, climbing, water sports
  - supplemental travel insurance, travel health insurance, and medical evacuation insurance
- Signs and symptoms for which care should be sought immediately
  - pelvic or abdominal pain, bleeding, fainting (ectopic pregnancy/miscarriage)
  - nausea, vomiting, abdominal bloating, shortness of breath, dehydration (OHSS)
  - symptoms of potential deep vein thrombosis or pulmonary embolism (unusual swelling of leg with pain in calf or thigh, unusual shortness of breath)
- Recommendations
  - immunizations based on risk assessment and up-to-date guideline
  - malaria prophylaxis, if indicated
  - preventive measures to decrease the above risks
- Paperwork
  - check airline and cruise line policies
  - letter confirming fitness to travel
  - copy of medical records (issue of confidentiality to be considered with the IVF patient)
  - letter for customs regarding medications (regulation regarding travelling with medications/needles)
  - ensure sufficient medication to cover entire duration of trip and possible delays
  - drug storage/refrigeration
  - time adjustment/effect of crossing time zones with drug administration
  - exemption letter or waiver for required vaccines

Pregnancy issues, if applicable
- Preparing for obstetric care (if becomes pregnant and embarking on long-term travel)
  - check coverage by medical insurance
  - arrange travel insurance, and medical evacuation insurance
  - arrange for obstetric care at destination

Continued

TABLE 20.2 (*Continued*)

Pre-Travel Consultation Checklist for the IVF Patient Traveller

- Comfort arrangements
  - comfortable clothing
  - bottled water
  - lighten itinerary if not accustomed to planned activities
- Postpone travel if risks outweigh benefits

Source: Adapted from Carroll D, Advising Travelers with Specific Needs: Pregnant Travelers. In: Brunette GW (Editor in Chief) *CDC Health Information for International Travel*, Chapter 8. Oxford University Press, 2014.

Potential contraindications to travel in the IVF patient may include:

1. OHSS: risk of thromboembolic disease, cardiorespiratory and renal compromise, inability to adopt the brace position in emergency landing due to enlarged ovaries and ascites with air travel
2. Early pregnancy complications: bleeding, abdominal pain, risk of miscarriage and ectopic pregnancy
3. Travel to potentially hazardous destinations:
   - High altitudes
   - Areas endemic for or with ongoing outbreaks of life-threatening food- or insect-borne infections
   - Areas where chloroquine-resistant *Plasmodium falciparum* malaria is endemic
   - Areas where live virus vaccines are required and recommended

What Immunizations Are Necessary and What Are the Risks?

Ideally, a woman should be up to date on routine vaccinations before embarking on IVF treatment. These are summarised in Tables 20.3A and B. The decision regarding whether to further vaccinate the IVF patient traveller depends on many factors including the destination, the duration of travel, the risk of contracting disease, the severity of the effect of the disease on the woman and the potential fetus, the adverse effects of the vaccine on her and/or the potential fetus and the risk perceptions of the woman and the healthcare provider. When considering whether to vaccinate an IVF patient for travel purposes the following guidelines may be helpful:

1. Check current vaccination status.
2. Follow up-to-date guidelines:
   - Ensure routine immunizations are up to date (e.g. tetanus and diphtheria boosters)
   - Consider if any immunizations are required (e.g. yellow fever in tropical Americas and Africa, quadrivalent meningitis vaccination prior to Hajj pilgrimage in Saudi Arabia); travellers to these countries who have contraindications should carry exemption documentation

TABLE 20.3A

Recommendations for Travel and IVF Patient*

Routinely Recommended Vaccine	Recommendation	Comments
Hepatitis	Recommended if otherwise indicated	
Hepatitis B	Recommended in some circumstances	
Human papillomavirus	Not recommended	
Influenza (inactivated)	Recommended	Inactivated
Influenza (LAIV)	Contraindicated	Live-attenuated vaccine
MMR	Contraindicated	Live-attenuated vaccine
MCV4 (MenACWY)	May be used if otherwise indicated	
PCV13	Inadequate data for specific recommendation	
PPSV23	Inadequate data for specific recommendation	
Polio	May be used if needed	Inactivated vaccine
Td	Should be used if otherwise indicated	
Tdap	Recommended	
Varicella	Contraindicated	
Zoster	Contraindicated	

Source: Adapted from CDC Guidelines for Vaccinating Pregnant Women: Abstracted from recommendation of the Advisory Committee on Immunization Practices (ACIP) April 2013.

TABLE 20.3B

Recommendations for Travel and IVF Patient

Travel and Other Vaccines	Recommendation	Comments
Anthrax	Low risk of exposure – not recommended	
	High risk of exposure – may be used	
BCG	Contraindicated	
Japanese Encephalitis	Inadequate data for specific recommendation	
MPSV4	May be used if otherwise indicated	Meningococcal quadrivalent polysaccharide vaccine (Menommune), meningococcal quadrivalent conjugate vaccine (Menactra)
Rabies (inactivated vaccine)	May be used if otherwise indicated	Imovax (human diploid cell vaccine), Rabavert (purified chick embryo cell), Verorab (purified Vero cell vaccine)

Continued

TABLE 20.3B (*Continued*)

Recommendations for Travel and IVF Patient

Travel and Other Vaccines	Recommendation	Comments
Typhoid	Inadequate data for specific recommendation (oral typhoid vaccine [Ty21a])	Inactivated injectable vaccine preferred (Typhim Vi, Typherix)
Smallpox	Pre-exposure – contraindicated Post-exposure – recommended	
Yellow fever (live-attenuated vaccine)	May be used if benefit outweighs risk	Recommended if true exposure unavoidable; postponement of travel to area of risk preferred
Pneumococcal vaccine (Pneumovax 23, Pneumo 23)	May be used if benefit outweighs risk	Inactivated vaccine
Tick-borne encephalitis vaccine (FSME-IMMUN Vaccine)	Insufficient data to comment on the use in pregnancy	
Oral cholera vaccine (Dukoral)	Indicated if the risk of the disease clearly outweighs the potential risk of the vaccine	Inactivated vaccine

Source: Adapted from CDC Guidelines for Vaccinating Pregnant Women: Abstracted from recommendation of the Advisory Committee on Immunization Practices (ACIP) April 2013.

3. Recommended immunizations are based upon the risk of exposure during the traveller's planned itinerary and current immune status (e.g. hepatitis A, typhoid, rabies, Japanese B encephalitis).

4. Ensure there is no contra-indication.

5. Recommended intervals between doses and vaccines should be followed to allow optimal antibody production prior to travel.

The evidence available to guide the safety of vaccination in pregnant women is based largely on reports of outcome after inadvertent use. The major organisations which provide recommendations, including the Centres for Disease Control and Prevention (CDC), WHO, the American Congress of Obstetricians and Gynaecologists (ACOG), the American Advisory Committee on Immunization Practices (ACIP) and the Canadian National Advisory Committee on Immunization (NACI), are largely in agreement with regard to immunization recommendations in pregnant women. No evidence exists of risk to the fetus from vaccinating pregnant women with inactivated virus or bacterial vaccines or toxoids. Live vaccines administered to a pregnant woman pose a theoretical risk to the fetus; therefore live-attenuated virus and live bacterial vaccines generally are contraindicated during pregnancy.

In general it is considered that the benefits of vaccinating pregnant women usually outweigh potential risks when the likelihood of disease exposure is high, when infection would pose a risk to the mother or fetus, and when the vaccine is unlikely to cause harm.[3]

What Steps Are Necessary to Avoid Malaria?

Malaria can be serious in the non-immune and much more so in the pregnant than in the semi-immune and non-pregnant woman. Heavy parasitaemia, severe anaemia, and sometimes profound hypoglycaemia may characterise malaria in pregnancy. This may be complicated by cerebral malaria and acute respiratory distress syndrome. Placental sequestration of parasites may result in fetal loss or miscarriage. An infant born to an infected mother is at increased risk of low birth weight and, although rare, congenital malaria.

Because no prophylactic regimen provides complete protection, the IVF patient should defer travel to malaria-endemic areas, particularly to areas with risk of acquisition of drug-resistant *Plasmodium falciparum* malaria. However, if travel cannot be avoided, special care should be taken to avoid mosquito bites, and use of an effective chemoprophylactic regimen is essential. In view of the potential for pregnancy, it will make sense to use the same drug regime recommended in pregnancy, particularly during organogenesis (first trimester).

Which Antimalarial Prophylactics Are Advised?

Chloroquine is the drug of choice for pregnant women for destinations with chloroquine-sensitive malaria and mefloquine for chloroquine-resistant malaria. Doxycycline is contraindicated because of the effects of the tetracyclines on the fetus after the fourth month of gestation, including bone growth inhibition and discoloration and dysplasia of teeth. Primaquine causes haemolytic anaemia in glucose-6-phosphate dehydrogenase (G6PD) deficiency. It is contraindicated in pregnancy because the fetus cannot be tested for G6PD deficiency. Atovaquone-proguanil (Malarone) is not generally recommended because of lack of available safety data (Table 20.4). Up-to-date recommendations on antimalarial drug use during pregnancy should be checked with CDC, RCOG (Royal College of Obstetricians and Gynaecologists) and relevant local authorities.[4–6]

The choice of chemoprophylaxis depends on specific incidence of malaria at the destination and level of drug resistance to *P. falciparum*. Specialist advice should be sought for women in the first trimester because of the small theoretical potential for teratogenicity from antimalarial drugs that must be weighed against the substantial risk of acquiring malaria. To avoid bites in a malaria-endemic area, the IVF patient should always sleep under treated mosquito nets, wear long clothing after dark that is impregnated with pyrethroid insecticide (permethrin) and use an effective mosquito repellent that contains DEET (N,N-diethyl-M-tolumide) in concentrations of 30% or less, which could be applied to clothing and the exposed parts of the skin.[7]

Communicable (Infectious) Diseases

Travel to many developing countries puts the IVF patient at increased risk of exposure to communicable diseases, some of which may manifest themselves more severely if pregnancy ensues. Travellers' diarrhoea affects 10–60% of visitors to tropical and semi-tropical regions of the developing world. Decreased gastric activity and slowed intestinal transit make the pregnant woman more vulnerable to severe dehydration

TABLE 20.4A

Malarial Chemoprophylaxis

Malarial chemoprophylaxis (if travel unavoidable)	Recommendation	Comments
Chloroquine or hydroxychloroquine	Drug of choice in chloroquine-sensitive areas	
Doxycycline	Not recommended	Adverse effects on the fetus with the use of tetracyclines when used after the fourth month of pregnancy, including discoloration and dysplasia of the teeth and inhibition of bone growth
Atovaquone-proguanil combination (malarone)	Limited data available to recommend use	Might be considered after careful discussion of the benefits and risks in women who cannot avoid travel to mefloquine-resistant areas
Mefloquine	Drug of choice for travel to chloroquine-resistant malaria areas	Recommended for use any time during pregnancy in chloroquine-resistant areas
Primaquine		Not recommended, as the G6PD status of the fetus cannot be established and the drug can be passed transplacentally

TABLE 20.4B

Miscellaneous Measures

Personal protection measures	Insect repellents with N,N-diethyl-M-tolumide (DEET) and insecticide-treated bed nets for sleeping should be used to reduce exposure to insect-borne diseases.
Air travel	Avoid travel if OHSS and/or early pregnancy problem (e.g. bleeding, pain, pregnancy of unknown location). Thromboprophylaxis as per up-to-date guideline (e.g. support stockings, leg movements, LMWH).
Motion sickness	Scopolamine patches should be avoided in pregnancy. Seabands are safe in pregnancy Phenothiazines including chlorpromazine (Largactil), prochlorperazine (Stemetil), and promethazine (Phenergan) can be used to prevent and treat motion sickness if necessary.
Traveller's diarrhoea	Loperamide (Imodium) may be used when necessary. Bismuth subsalicylate compounds are contraindicated. Azithromycin is the drug of first choice to treat traveller's diarrhoea. Third-generation cephalosporins can be used. Fluoroquinolones are generally contraindicated in pregnancy.

and ketosis. When advising IVF patients on how best to avoid contracting infectious diseases when travelling overseas, the following guidance should be given:

1. Strict hand hygiene and food and water precautions should be stressed.[8]

2. Bottled or boiled water is preferable to chemically treated or filtered water. Iodine-containing compounds should not be used to purify water for pregnant women because of potential effects on the fetal thyroid with prolonged use.[9]

3. The treatment of choice for travellers' diarrhoea is prompt and vigorous oral hydration (oral rehydration salts mixed with filtered water, which is safe in pregnancy). Use a sugary drink if oral rehydration salts are not available, because sugars are likely to increase water absorption.

4. Early recourse to parenteral rehydration is advised if the patient does not respond to oral fluids.

If the patient does not respond, consider treatment for atypical pathogens after confirmed diagnosis on a stool sample; check safety of specific antibiotics in pregnancy. Azithromycin may be given to pregnant women if clinically indicated. Bismuth subsalicylate is contraindicated because of the theoretical risks of fetal bleeding from salicylates and teratogenicity from the bismuth.

Food-borne illnesses of particular concern during pregnancy include toxoplasmosis and listeriosis. The infection may cross the placenta and cause spontaneous miscarriage, stillbirth, or congenital infection. The patient should therefore be warned to avoid unpasteurised cheeses and undercooked meat products.

Parasitic diseases are less common but may cause concern, particularly in women who are visiting developing parts of the world. Intestinal helminthes rarely cause illness severe enough to warrant treatment during pregnancy, and most can safely be addressed with symptomatic treatment when the pregnancy is over.

Protozoan intestinal infections, such as with *Giardia*, *Entamoeba histolytica*, and *Cryptosporidium*, may cause acute gastroenteritis and chronic malabsorption, resulting in fetal growth restriction. *Entamoeba histolytica* may cause invasive disease, including amoebic liver abscess and colitis. Pregnant women are advised to avoid swimming or wading in freshwater lakes, streams, and rivers that may harbor schistosomes. These protozoan infections often do require treatment in pregnancy. Hepatitis A and E are both spread by the feco-oral route and could be associated with significant perinatal morbidity and mortality.

The absorption of oral medications, such as oestradiol for frozen embryo cycle, may be affected by gastroenteritis. Appropriate measures should be in place, such as repeating the dose shortly after vomiting or increasing the dose in case of profuse diarrhoea.

Air Travel

If possible, the IVF patient should avoid air travel until the outcome of treatment is known and any immediate complications such as OHSS have resolved.

In the case of the potentially pregnant IVF patient, specific concerns have been raised about the safety of air travel during pregnancy.

TABLE 20.5

Recommendations to Reduce the Risk of DVT

- Use aisle seat if possible to facilitate movement
- Mobilise throughout flight – every 30 minutes
- Avoid dehydration
- Increase water but limit caffeine and alcohol intake
- Consider graduated elastic compression stockings for flights longer than 4 hours
- Consider low molecular weight heparin in the presence of additional risk factors for DVT

Venous thromboembolism is 10 times more common in pregnant women than in matched non-pregnant counterparts, and it complicates about 1 in 1000 pregnancies.[10] Inherent prothrombotic changes of pregnancy and ovarian stimulation, and in particular hCG (human chorionic gonadotrophin) administration, may contribute to this. Travel may confer further risk because of immobility, low oxygen tension, and low humidity, which lead to venous stasis and dehydration.[11,12]

Recommendations to reduce the risk of DVT are summarised in Table 20.5.

Exposure to Radiation

Older airport security machines are magnetometers and are not harmful to the fetus. Newer security machines use backscatter x-ray scanners, which emit low levels of radiation; most experts agree that the risk of radiation exposure from these scanners is extremely low.

The risk of adverse effects to the fetus from radiation during a single flight is negligible, but pregnant women who are frequent fliers, and airline staff who fly, may reach levels of exposure over the recommended maximum.[13] The radiation exposure from a 10-hour flight is estimated to be 0.05 mSv.[14] Guidelines for diagnostic imaging in pregnancy from the ACOG conclude that there is no known increase in fetal malformations or miscarriage or effects on growth at levels less than 50 mSv.[15]

A meta-analysis has reported that the risk of pregnancy loss is significantly greater in flight attendants than in controls (odds ratio 1.62, 95% confidence interval 1.29 to 2.04).[16] However, it is unclear whether this increased risk is related to increased exposure to radiation or some other factor associated with frequent high-altitude air travel.

Sporting Activities

The IVF patient should be discouraged from undertaking unaccustomed vigorous physical activity. Trauma to enlarged ovaries could be catastrophic. Swimming and snorkelling during pregnancy are generally safe, but waterskiing can result in falls that inject water into the birth canal. Most experts advise against scuba diving for pregnant women because of the risk of fetal gas embolism during decompression, which may travel to the brain, causing ischemia and hypoxia. There are no good data to confirm or refute an increased risk of birth defects from diving. Pregnant female divers have been exposed to hyperbaric oxygen therapy for decompression illness (DCI), and there have been no reports of ill effects on the fetus; therefore pregnant women who suffer from DCI can be treated this way just as non-pregnant divers. Previous diving prior to the discovery of a pregnancy is not per se an absolute indication for termination, as data has failed to show teratogenic risk in humans.[17]

Environmental Considerations

The general advice regarding environmental considerations in pregnancy could apply to the IVF patient traveller.

Air pollution may pose more health problems during pregnancy because mucus production is increased and ciliary clearance of the bronchial tree is slowed. Body temperature regulation is not as efficient during pregnancy, and extremes of temperature may harm the fetus. Vasovagal events such as fainting may result from the vasodilatory effect of a hot environment. For these reasons, accommodation should be sought in air-conditioned quarters and activities restricted in hot environments. Pregnant women should avoid activities at high altitude unless trained for and accustomed to such activities. The common symptoms of acute mountain sickness (insomnia, headache, and nausea) are also frequently associated with pregnancy and some with OHSS, and this may pose diagnostic difficulty. According to the CDC, all pregnant women should avoid altitudes >3,658 meters (>12,000 feet). In addition, altitudes >2,500 meters (>8,200 feet) should be avoided in late or high-risk pregnancy.[18] Although compelling reasons to use acetazolamide may exist, most experts recommend simply a slower ascent with adequate time for acclimatisation. Probably the largest concern regarding high-altitude travel in pregnancy is that many high-altitude destinations are inaccessible and far from medical care.

Key Management Points

1. Ideally, international travel should not be undertaken by the IVF patient until the outcome of treatment is known.
2. Pre-travel evaluation with a healthcare professional/travel clinic, preferably with input from her fertility and other relevant medical specialist, should take place if travel is necessary.
3. Risk assessment to enable an individualised best package of management should be put in place.
4. Measures should be taken to prevent or at least reduce the risk of communicable or infectious diseases and appropriate measures for prompt management if symptoms develop.
5. Generally, the benefits of vaccinating the IVF patient outweigh the potential risks when the likelihood of disease exposure is high, the infection is likely to pose a risk to the woman (and the potential fetus), and the vaccine is unlikely to cause harm.
6. Malaria avoidance measures as well as effective and appropriate chemoprophylaxis should be in place when travelling to malaria-endemic parts of the world.
7. Ensuring compliance with policies and regulations as a special traveller and obtaining appropriate travel and medical insurance should be part and parcel of the planning process.

REFERENCES

1. World Health Organisation (WHO). International Travel and Health (ITH 2012 Edition).
2. Spira AM. Preparing the traveller. *Lancet.* 2003 Apr 19; 361(9366):1368–81.
3. General recommendations on immunization: recommendations of the Advisory Committee on Immunization Practices (ACIP). *MMWR Morb Mortal Wkly Rep.* 2011; 60(No. 2):26.
4. Arguin PM, Tan KR. *Infectious Diseases Related to Travel: Malaria.* Atlanta, GA: Centers for Disease Control and Prevention, 2013, Table 3-10 and Chapter 3.
5. Royal College of Obstetricians and Gynaecologists (RCOG). *The Prevention of Malaria in Pregnancy.* Greentop Guideline No. 54A. London: RCOG; 2010.
6. Expert centres in the UK on malarial chemoprophylaxis:
   Malaria Reference Laboratory. http://www.malaria-reference.co.uk.
   National Travel Health Network and Centre. http://www.nathnac.org.
   Liverpool School of Tropical Medicine. http://www.liv.ac.uk/lstm.
   TRAVAX: The A–Z of Healthy Travel (Health Protection Scotland and NHS Scotland). http://www.travax.nhs.uk.
7. Nasci RS, Zielinski-Gutierrez E, Wirtz RA, et al. *Protection against Mosquitoes, Ticks, and Other Insects and Arthropods.* CDC Health Information for International Travel 2014 (The Yellow Book) Centers for Disease Control and Prevention and Gary W. Brunette. Chapter 2 The Pre-Travel Consultation Counselling & Advice for Travelers.
8. Watson JC, Hlavsa MC, Griffin PM. *Food and Water Precautions.* CDC Health Information for International Travel 2014 (The Yellow Book) Centers for Disease Control and Prevention and Gary W. Brunette. Chapter 2 The Pre-Travel Consultation Counselling & Advice for Travelers.
9. Backer HD. *Water Disinfection for Travelers.* CDC Health Information for International Travel 2014 (The Yellow Book) Centers for Disease Control and Prevention and Gary W. Brunette. Chapter 2 The Pre-Travel Consultation Counselling & Advice for Travelers.
10. Rodger MA, Walker M, Wells PS. Diagnosis and treatment of venous thromboembolism in pregnancy. *Best Pract Res Clin Haematol.* 2003; 16:279–96.
11. Royal College of Obstetricians and Gynaecologists, London. Air Travel and Pregnancy. Scientific Advisory Committee Paper, 2008. http://www.rcog.org.uk/womens-health/clinical-guidance/air-travel-and-pregnancy.
12. WRIGHT project (WHO Research into Global Hazards of Air Travel). *Final Report of Phase I.* Geneva: World Health Organization.
13. Magann EF, Chauhan SP, Dahlke JD, et al. Air travel and pregnancy outcomes: A review of pregnancy regulations and outcomes for passengers, flight attendants and aviators. *Obstet Gynaecol Surv.* 2010; 5:396–402.
14. ACOG Committee on Obstetric Practice. ACOG Committee Opinion. Number 299. Guidelines for diagnostic imaging during pregnancy. *Obstet Gynecol.* 2004; 104:647–51.
15. Barish R. In-flight radiation exposure during pregnancy. *Obstet Gynecol.* 2004; 103:1326–30.
16. Advising on travel during pregnancy. *BMJ.* 2011; 342:d2506.
17. Fife CE, Fife WP. Should pregnant women scuba dive? *J Travel Med.* 1994; 1:160–5.
18. Centers for Disease Control and Prevention. *CDC Health Information for International Travel 2010.* Atlanta, GA: Department of Health and Human Services, Public Health Service, 2009.

Index